ISBN 978-0-282-48808-6
PIBN 10853525

# SUPERB VIRILITY OF MANHOOD

*Giving the Causes and Simple Home Methods of Curing the Weaknesses of Men*

BY

BERNARR MACFADDEN

Assisted by Various Medical and Other Authorities

PUBLISHED BY

PHYSICAL CULTURE PUBLISHING CO.

PHYSICAL CULTURE CITY, SPOTSWOOD P. O., N. J.

12 AND 13 RED LION COURT, FLEET STREET
LONDON, ENGLAND
Printed in U. S. A.

# CONTENTS.

CONTENTS

CHAPTER XXXIX

ABBREVIATED GENERAL INSTRUCTIONS

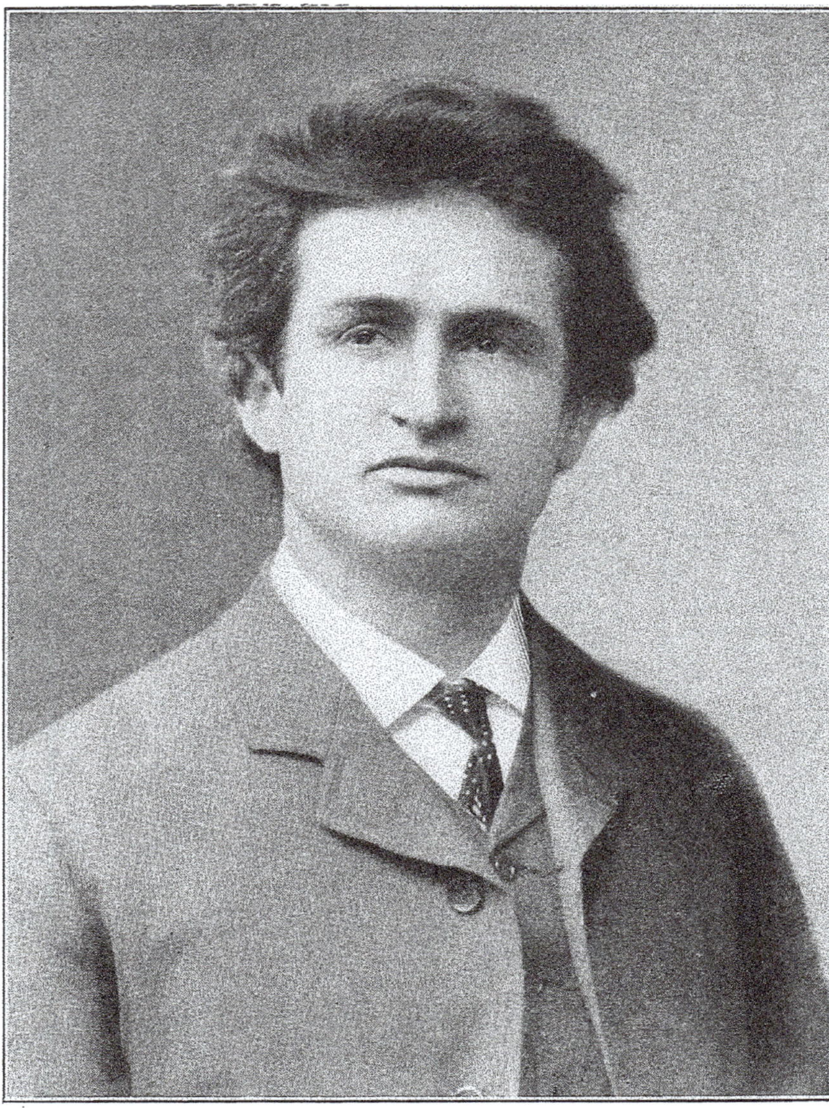

*Yours for Health*
*Bernarr Macfadden*

# PREFACE

This book is for men. It talks plainly on subjects of vital importance to men. The evils of to-day which are the result of the present conventional prudishness can only be remedied by knowledge.

Prudery and prurient mystery cover a multitude of evils. They are responsible for the greater part of the physical degeneracy of the human race. This book has been written to lift the veil in which they insist on shrouding subjects of the utmost importance to humanity. Knowledge is power, and for sufferers from the diseases which are discussed in this volume, the knowledge here given, is of monumental value.

Without virile manhood, the male of the human species is indeed to be pitied. And there are thousands on thousands of weak and suffering men who call for added pity because, through no fault of their own, they are ignorant of the fact that they can be benefited and permanently cured of their maladies by the common sense methods the writer so emphatically advocates, but which, alas! are so little known to the greater public.

There has been enough of quackery and mystery in relation to the topics with which this book deals. Let the blackness of ignorance be dispelled by the brilliant rays of knowledge to illumine the path that leads to safe, sensible and sane cures for sexual troubles.

The following pages contain all the information it is possible for the writer to give on each subject. Everything of value that was obtainable and appertained to the book as a whole has been clearly stated here. We have nothing further to sell, no further information to give. If you are a sufferer and possess ordinary intelligence, a careful study of this work should enable you to prescribe a course for yourself that should insure you a cure.

The writer in some cases gives individual advice but his charges for so doing are by no means small. He considers his time given to individual consultations worth far more than that of high-priced physicians. As a rule he has found that those who want special advice have neglected to study the theories of the cure pertinent to their cases. If you will conscientiously study your complaint with the assistance of this book you will finally become able to answer your own questions. So that you are then the possessor of conclusions that are yours through some amount of work, and it is far better for you if you prepare yourself for remedying your trouble in this selfsame manner.

Bernarr Macfadden

# CHAPTER I

## WOES OF WEAK MEN

Pitiable Condition of the Victims of Their Own or Their Parents' Sexual Excesses.

That which beauty of feature, form and character is to a woman, strength of mind and body is to a man. Each is in turn the distinctive characteristic of the sex which it adorns. Unlike, the two qualities are yet essential to each other, and the ultimate of human happiness is to be found in the presence of their union when it takes the shape of a marriage of hearts and hands. The mating instinct is the most powerful of all the instincts of humanity, and upon it are based every institution of our race. The home apart from its personal aspects is the fountain of national life, the source of national virtues and the conservator of national greatness. But homes, in the actual sense of the word, are not possible unless they who make them are possessed of the primal, the peculiar qualities of their respective sexes. And of such, that of the man — vigor or strength — is the more necessary of the two.

Mere facial beauty may be wanting in a woman, but she can atone for its absence by charms of form or by being the owner of that mysterious and attractive gift which we know as "femininity." Some of the most famous women of history were not remarkable for beauty of feature. On the other hand it is only strong men that have left their impress on the ages.

The fact is that the weak man is an anomaly. He has, either through his own or by reason of his parents' actions, defeated the purposes of his creation, one of the chiefest of which is the procreation of his kind. His sallow cheeks, shrivelled muscles, lustreless eyes, scanty breath and all the rest of it, tell of a physique which is either incapable of, or can only indifferently perform the sacred duties of a husband. Apart from that, the weak man is terribly handicapped in the struggle for existence as far as material things are concerned. It may be that he need not trouble over financial affairs. In that case he is in a sense fortunate, although he can never be truly happy. But these lucky ones are not plentiful and so the majority of the unhappy creatures muddle through life, overtaken and thrust aside by the strong, pitied by some, despised by others, a source of misery to themselves and the cause of regret and discomfort to those with whom they are associated.

"From the physiologist's and the utilitarian's standpoints the weakling has no place in the internal economy of a community. He is a danger to the physical well-being of his fellows and a drag on their material progress. If he marries he is likely to transmit his mental and physical shortcomings to his descendants in an ever-widening circle of degenerative evils. As he cannot bear his full burden of the toils of life it follows that someone else has to shoulder added responsibilities. He radiates an atmosphere of depression and lack of vitality. Fortunately, nature limits his powers for harm by cutting short his days or in many cases, by rendering him incapable of repeating himself in a sickly progeny."—*Christopher Weldon, M.D.*

The highest, and the noblest joys of life are, as intimated, to be found in the well balanced unions of the sexes. From these relations the unfortunate victim of heredity or excesses is forever barred. Women usually retain the first instinct of sex much more strongly than men do. So that a normal girl in selecting a mate insists on that, in him, which she possesses in a lesser degree—strength; the strength of body which shall protect her from physical harm, the strength of character which shall guarantee his faithfulness and her happiness, the strength of will and purpose which shall insure her and her children a home and a strength of sexual powers which will richly gratify her maternal instincts.

Now woman's intuitions warn her that the weak man is the owner of neither one or the other of these types of strength; at least, in a well developed form, that a marriage with him would mean a marriage in name only, and that misery, disappointment and repulsion must follow on the union as surely as night follows day. Physically weak, he must therefore be sexually weak, and weakness of character is always found in company with the other weaknesses named. It is true that as long as there are women who will marry for money, for any sort of home, for sickly sentiment or for mistaken motives of pity, so long will these alleged men be permitted to contract unions that are libels on the word marriage. But for the most part the wholesome minded female will shrink with horror from such an alliance. Perhaps, when the world is wiser and realizes to the full its responsibilities to itself and posterity, it will forbid any man or woman inflicting on that posterity those evils which are the fruits of shattered constitutions, and resultant impaired vitality.

"What is decided among animals by force is adjudged among civilized men by law or reason. Yet in some cases it would almost seem as if the brutes were wiser than we, especially in those matters that relate to the preservation of the health and strength of their species. A lion or stag, for instance, must prove their claims to be fathers of their kind by overcoming weaker rivals. These combats among the males of all wild animals may suggest cruelty on the part of

Nature but they answer their purpose most effectively — that of weeding out the weak ones. As a result, an animal in a state of Nature is as nearly perfect physically as a created being can be.

But with us there is absolutely no safeguard against racial degeneracy. Even that feminine instinct that makes a woman revolt at the idea of a union with one of the other sex who is inferior to her, mentally or physically, has been blunted by social custom or disuse. Among savages a marriageable girl looks with disdain upon a suitor who is lacking in those distinctive attributes of a MAN — strength or courage. But with us it is different and otherwise. The rickety, nerveless, flabby-muscled products of the like parents and artificial environments of civilization are allowed to marry without let or hindrance. If the dream of Carlyle in his Sartor Resartus could but come true and people wore no clothes whatever, we should have an effective object lesson on the folly of permitting men and women to marry who are wanting in the first qualities needed by the matrimonial relation. And contra-wise the soundness of the 'savage' principle is exemplified by the superb physical proportions of, say, a tribe of Zulus or Ingorettes."—*B. J. Lawson, M.D.*

Not only is the weak man deprived of the lasting comfort and profound happiness that are bred from the love and embraces of a healthy, congenial wife, but in addition, he is prevented from living his youth over again in the persons of his children. No small proportion of family joys arise from this same rejuvenation of the parents in their offspring. If he has little ones, he will assuredly learn how certain it is that the sins of the parents are visited on the children. For weakness is a sin against the body that was intended to be strong. And if he has the remnants of a conscience or the traces of a heart he will curse the day when he caused the conception of the puny, pain-wracked little creatures who have the misfortune to call him father.

But he is not merely barred from the solaces of matrimony. The possessor of that superb health and strength which the Almighty intended should be as common to humanity as air itself, has joy in the mere act of living — a joy that is more than a joy, an exhilaration of body and heart and soul, that is positively intoxicating. The full tide of vitality sweeps through the being of such a man in resistless fashion, and he in turn feels himself resistless when it comes to accomplishing the things on which he has set his mind or heart. Work to this man is recreation, exercise of any kind the cause of added happiness and he courts difficulties for the sake of the sheer satisfaction of overcoming them. In love, an irresistible wooer; in business, a notable success; in combat, a conqueror, he proves the possibilities of a man as God planned man to be.

Contrast him with the weak man. The daily existence of the latter is a round of physical discomforts and mental disturbances. He eats, knowing that his digestive organs will fail in their duty. He shrinks from a petty amount of physical effort, being assured that he will pay for it in laboring lungs, a palpitating heart and trembling limbs. He dreads mental toil because of the racking nervous headaches that will follow. He shuns the society of his kind, his days are filled with shadowy forebodings and his nights with broken and feverish slumbers. He knows not of the delights of a plunge into a pool fed by mountain streams or of cresting the long rollers of the surf. The pleasures of the gymnasium, the links, the saddle, the shell, the spray-sprinkled deck, or rod or gun, snowshoe or ski, are all sealed to him. He can hardly be said to live, he vegetates like some of the lower forms of animal life only he is less happy than they. If he survives to that age when a man's main comfort are his memories, he is the more unhappy because his memories are those of excesses for which he has paid dearly and the sorrow and suffering that he has inflicted on himself and others by reason of such. That these excesses were due to temperament, ignorance or heredity does not affect the results. Offended Nature demands her price from the offender and she invariably gets it.

Yet Nature is a merciful mother after all. If the violator of her laws turns to her and asks her help in restoring to him his manhood and the many things that manhood means, she rarely refuses him her aid. But she insists that her means and methods shall be used and followed implicitly. And these are simple enough. Everything that builds the body of the child on healthful lines, will also build the body of the weak man into renewed health if the work be done under intelligent direction. Diet, exercise, ventilation, the bath, and so forth, are the factors in the restoration of strength and vitality. And if humanity could be induced to replace the pills and powders and potions of the doctors with those factors, that most pitiable object under Heaven — the muscularly, sexually, morally weak man would quickly become extinct and nothing remain of him but a contemptuous memory.

# CHAPTER II

## MISTAKES OF MEDICAL MEN

### Mainly Due to the Manner in Which They Ignore Nature's Plain Promptings.

"If medical science were a positive science as is mathematics and its professors, able to apply its principles to daily life with the certainty of geometrical propositions, it would be folly to do otherwise than accept any medical opinion of established authority with entire confidence. This, however, is not the case, and members of the medical profession would be the last to lay claim to it."—*E. Blackwell, M.D.*

The general truth of the cynical maxim that "a doctor is one who pours drugs of which he knows little into a body of which he knows less," has never been questioned by thinking men and women and is admitted by members of the medical profession themselves when no patients are around or fees in sight. Read any of the publications devoted to the doings of the doctors and it will be found that a " practice " rests on a foundation composed of two thirds hide-bound tradition and one third experiment. Some few physicians have had the courage to break away from the old order of things and adopt curative methods that are identical with those used by physical culturists. It may be added that such men are among the most prominent and successful of their profession before the public to-day. But the great majority of their fellows blunder along in the good old fashion, burying but not profiting by their mistakes except to the extent of the bills paid by the surviving relatives.

No better illustration of the stupidly illogical methods of our medical "schools" can be obtained than that furnished by the " general practitioner " when his patient is suffering from, say, loss of manly vigor and vitality. In nine cases out of ten such a patient is paying the penalty of some form of sexual excess. But in any event his bodily organs refuse to perform their functions, he is debilitated generally, his mental powers are more or less affected, his nervousness is excessive and in short, he bears all the ear marks of a man who has overdrawn so terribly on his vitality that his account is pretty nearly closed.

Does the doctor ask from whence and how did his patient get his original stock of vitality and does he try to replenish the exhausted supply at that same source? Does he reflect that only like breeds like and that in consequence you may just as well try to hatch a lobster from a liver pill as to attempt to obtain vitality from drugs? Does he understand that the patient's habits have in all likelihood charged his bloed with impurities and that the first step to recovery must be the elimination of them by natural means? Does he realize that before nutritive food can be given to any extent, the digestive organs must be capable of assimilating such food? Not a bit of it.

"You are badly run down," says the man of medicine. "You want a thorough rest, a generous diet — plenty of rare beef, you know — and take this tonic three times a day. See me a week hence and let me know how you are getting on."

The patient obeys and one of two things follows. There is crape on the door of the late sufferer at an early date, or crape at a date deferred. It depends on the power of the remaining vitality of the unfortunate to stand off the results of the treatment. But the crape is inevitable sooner or later. The tonic — always a modified poison — makes a further drain on the vitality by reason of the efforts of the body to get rid of it. The "generous" diet, including the bloody meat, proving too "generous" for the enfeebled digestive organs, is not assimilated and so ferments and produces peptones, virulent poisons which remain in and further pollute the blood. The " thorough rest " deprives the sufferer of the exercise which would have helped his system to throw off its foulness through perspiration, the increased action of the lungs and excretory organs and have aided his clogged digestive apparatus to resume its functions.

In other words the perhaps well-meaning, but certainly mistaken " general practitioner," has misused one of the factors in restoring lost vigor, that is, diet; has totally ignored another, which is exercise; and has further poisoned an already poisoned system by prescribing tonics.

Apart from errors in the actual treatment of weakened victims of sexual passions, grave mistakes are often made by doctors in diagnosing the cases of such. The consequences of these blunders are of a disastrous nature. Listen to what a famous authority on the subject has to say about them:

"The pathological results of venereal excess are now all well known. But the gradual derangements of health experienced by its victims are not at first recognized by them, and even physicians may take the symptoms to be the beginning of very different diseases. How often symptoms are considered as cases of hypochondria or chronic gastritis or the commencement of heart disease which are really the results of some form of generative abuse. A general exhaustion of the whole physical force; symptoms of cerebral congestion; or paralysis wrongly attributed to some cerebro-spinal lesion are often due to the same causes. The same may be said of some of the severest forms of insanity. Many cases of consumption appearing in young men who have no hereditary tendency to the disease enter into the same category. So many diseases are vainly treated by medical men which are really caused by abuse of these important functions of the body."—*Professor Michel Levy.*

In other words many doctors are incapable of recognizing the results of the loss of vitality even when they are brought into contact with them. And what is worse they are liable to treat the patient for an imaginary disease, thereby not only aggravating the actual trouble, but in addition putting a further burden on the already over-burdened constitution. If a healthy man were to be dosed with drugs that he positively didn't need, he would probably be a sick man in a day or so. Imagine then the results of such drugs being unnecessarily poured into a system whose vitality, as it is, is barely sufficient to keep body and soul together!

The mischievous aftermath of a physician's blunders are mainly due to moss-covered superstitions. The "leech" of old times was a mixture of a quack, a magician and an alchemist. To impress his ignorant patients he administered to them powdered spiders, essence of bat's blood, burnt hair of murderers and other weird "drugs." The "leech" passed but his gulls go on forever. Yet the public still insists on its drugs and the "schools," seeing the expediency and profit of ministering to the popular demand for nasty tasting things in pills and bottles, desired not to throw a damper on the worship of the drug fetich. So, while the "leech" of today is a solemn, sleek gentleman who owns his own brougham and prescribes dear little sugar-coated pellets instead of desiccated frog's eyes, the principle is practically the same as in days of old. Nature's obvious and certain way of restoring health to a wrecked body is ignored by the multitude and instead, we have that same body charged with all manner of deleterious compounds. Then, as intimated, comes the aftermath.

Doctors blunder but Nature's curative method admits of no mistakes. Doctors have a score of alleged remedies for one malady, Nature but one cure for all ailments. Doctors admit that medical science is more or less empirical; Nature's aid to the stricken is as sure as it is safe. And Nature never makes an incorrect diagnosis.

# CHAPTER III

## PATENT MEDICINE FRAUDS

### Something About the Methods of a Most Dangerous Class of Criminals.

When a petty thief through the medium of false pretences, gets hold of your money, the machinery of justice is put into motion to the end of his being punished according to his deserts. And yet there are innumerable criminals in this country protected by the law and not infrequently rewarded by fortunes, who not only rob thousands of people of millions of money annually through representations of the most fraudulent but in addition, often deprive their dupes of life itself. These scoundrels are a certain class of patent medicine men, for the most part those who advertise that they have an infallible remedy for venereal diseases, lost manhood and lost vitality. Only the Recording Angel knows the amount of sorrow and suffering for which these vampires of their kind are responsible.

On the continent of Europe the power for evil of the patent medicine man is reduced to a minimum by statutes which are designed to protect the public from his callous greed. As an illustration of the severity of the laws governing him and his methods there, may be cited a recent case in Berlin in which the quack was sentenced to four years' imprisonment and ordered to pay a heavy fine for misrepresenting the ingredients of his nostrum and claiming for it virtues which it did not possess. If the German mode of dealing with these fellows became effective in this country the population of the penitentiaries would be vastly increased and the income of the judiciaries enlarged in proportion.

A famous English author once remarked

that "The population of Great Britain is nearly 60,000,000 — chiefly fools." In the same spirit, a notorious confidence man of America gave utterance to the adage that: "A sucker is born every minute." Also did not the late P. T. Barnum allege that the American public "loved to be humbugged."

It is on this credulity and ignorance of the masses that the patent medicine fakir trades and thrives. If it be asked why legislative action does not protect the people in this connection, the reply is that there is such a thing as a Patent Medicine Trust or Trusts which represent the investment of an enormous amount of capital, and that capital does pretty much as it likes in the matter of having laws made or unmade.

If it be further asked why the alleged champion and guardian of the rights of the community, the newspaper press, does not take up arms against these cold-blooded malefactors the answer can be found in the advertising columns of the newspapers. Patent medicine advertisements are big, usually permanent and invariably lucrative. It is not good business to publish "sensations" if they hit at your best customers you must remember. And besides that, the business department of a newspaper controls the editorial policy.

So it is that in one part of a newspaper a most scathing arraignment of some financial or commercial trust or of a man who is asserted to be a public enemy will appear, but in the same issue, under the head of advertisements, one can read seductive and insinuating offers to those suffering from "hidden weaknesses," etc., etc. The editors and managers may no doubt wonder how enough victims can be caught to pay for such large advertising bills, but somehow they seem to forget that these same victims are as capable of suffering as are those who are injured by the trusts, that are so bitterly denounced — all trusts except the Patent Medicine Trust. It is an indelible stain on the reputation of that magnificent profession, journalism, that the fragile, inexperienced, nervous wrecks of humanity, can be thus robbed, physically and financially, by quacks and should-be convicts, who hire the space and reputation of the most widely read newspapers and periodicals to assist them in the furtherance of their nefarious business.

Yet, unquestionably the use of patent medicines is declining. The public has been so deceived and robbed so brazenly and cruelly of money and health by these rank fakirs that it is beginning to lose faith in the ridiculous claims made by the proprietors of so-called remedies and specifics.

Some of these claims are so preposterous as to be absolutely funny. Others are based on an impudent assumption of the general lack of knowledge on the part of the public. In other instances the quack exhibits his own ignorance of many things including the English language. There is for example, a tremenduously advertised "Woman's Prescription" which, we are assured, consists of "botanic *and* vegetable substances." A "botanic" that wasn't some sort of a vegetable substance would be a curiosity. It is said that a half million of money was spent last year in giving publicity to a liquid which, so we are gravely informed, "contains all the elements of oxygen and when swallowed takes them to all parts of the body." As oxygen is a simple element in itself which can't possibly be split into other elements and, as every school boy knows, the body can only get its oxygen through the medium of the lungs, the fluent lying of this quack will be apparent. Still another arrant humbug plays the changes on the dear old restore-vitality-by-electricity fraud by announcing that he has an "electrically charged" water or something equivalent to it in which you bathe yourself and so absorb the " life-giving fluid." Again the average school boy can tell you that you can just as easily bottle sunbeams or fill a hole with quicksilver as persuade electricity to stop in water. Still another charlatan lays claim to something which will kill each, every and any sort of microbe. "All disease is due to microbes in your blood," says this ingenious gentleman. " My mixture will knock everyone of 'em cold in quick time. Why have disease then? Why die?" And yet in spite of this charmingly easy way of abolishing suffering and death, the mortality returns show no signs of diminution. The X-ray as a cure for cancer and allied diseases has been the subject of much careful experiment on the part of many prominent specialists and has been found to be more or less of a failure. But we have X-ray "institutes" galore where — so the proprietors claim — you can be relieved of everything, certainly of your money. The publicity given to the discovery of radium resulted in a heavy crop of radium fakes, all of which are alleged to cure anything from soft corns to hydrocephalus. And so the story goes. The quack columns of the newspapers do indeed vouch for the truth of Barnum's assertion.

Think of the vast sums annually spent for these various "remedies," which are supposed to bring back to the wasted victims of excesses the strength and virility which have been frittered away by them. The amount would almost pay the national debt. And do these "remedies" cure? Do they ever even benefit? Never! On the contrary they work infinite harm. The manufacturers of these base impositions no doubt profit by them, but no one else. If the evil ended with the mere fleecing of the unwary, the consequences would not be so serious, but thousands are buoyed with false hope after reading of the wonderful cures allegedly wrought by these frauds, and becoming imbued with the belief that these spurious remedies are the only available methods of cure, they take no steps to become interested in natural restorative means which would bring health and strength in every instance back to the sufferer where such a result is possible. But the dupes go on, year after year, trying one quack remedy after another, until the grave opens and ends their miseries.

No cry of murder goes up at the funeral of the victim of greed and misrepresentation. He is laid peacefully away with lamentations and regrets and Divine Providence is credited with his taking off. But who is to blame for this murder — this poisoning by slow degrees of a life that might have been useful and prolonged? That legalized homicide, the patent medicine man. Enumerate all the deaths that occur in a modern war through diseases and battles and multiply it by a hundred, and it would probably approximate the actual number of persons who annually lose their lives through quackery.

This shocking state of affairs will never be altered as long as the laws or rather want of laws, relative to patent medicine frauds remain as they are or until the public is better educated in those matters on which it is now so appallingly ignorant. If you are ever tempted to have any dealings with these blood-suckers reflect that their whole aim and effort is to extract as much money from their victim as possible and to this end it is their policy not to cure him, but to keep him sick as long as they conveniently can.

# CHAPTER IV

## ELECTRIC BELT HUMBUGS

### Gulling People in the Name of that of which They Know Nothing.

The " electric belt " fake while not quite so harmful as the swindles spoken of in the preceding chapter is nevertheless productive of dangerous consequences for the reason that it lulls the sufferer into a sense of false security, by impressing upon him the idea that he is " doing something " for his ailment. These electric belt fakirs are up to date. Nearly every one of their conspicuous advertisements contains artistically drawn figures of athletic men in a physical condition that could only be obtained by consistent and careful training. The inference of the advertisement is that a strip of leather or other material and a few bits of metal has brought into being the pictured Hercules. If one of these belts could work such a miracle of muscle there would, of course, be no further necessity for an athlete to make any preparation for a race or a pugilist for a contest. The weeks of arduous work in training quarters would be things of the past and instead, the intending competitors would strap an assortment of Dr. Tommyrot's belts around their limbs and bodies and simply loaf around watching their " wind " improve and their sinews harden in the meantime.

The brotherhood of quacks have much in common and so we find that the owners of these fakes make the same ridiculous claims for them as are made by patent-medicine vendors for their nostrums, namely, that diseases which in every case are brought about by the violation of the primal laws of health, can be remedied by the sufferer merely applying one of their belts to his person. According to their claims, there is no need for the patient to give the slightest attention to the cause of the trouble or to its results, since the belts will in every case produce the desired cure.

Some of these men, however, supplement the sale of their belts with advice of a semi-medical nature. If good results accrue, the belt is of course credited with the same. If it doesn't there is silence on the subject.

The truth is that electric belts never have and never can cure or assist in curing a disease of any kind whatever. Neither have they been of the smallest aid in restoring lost vitality. In some cases where the patient has had an imaginary disorder that could be remedied only by an appeal to the imagination — such cases are not rare — the belt has been of benefit if the sufferer was sufficiently impressed by the claims of its makers. But a peanut or a cobblestone would have been equally effective and a great deal less expensive if the patient could be persuaded into believing that they had " electric " curative powers also.

Charlatans and impostors of all sorts trade upon the ignorance of their victims. And when, as in the case of electricity, everybody knows that in which these impostors deal by name, but not by nature, the task of gulling the public is easy indeed. The truth of the matter is that after years of experiment with electricity as a curative agent, experts have come to no satisfactory conclusions regarding it. The best that can be said of it is, that it acts as a temporary muscular stimulant but only when properly applied and when the best apparatus is used. But that is all and to claim that it can " restore " lost vitality or cure a multitude of maladies is humbug of the most transparent.

More than that the belts are in themselves distinct frauds. They are supposed to generate electricity which passes into the body of the wearer. They do nothing of the kind. To create a current of electricity outside of a dynamo, a " battery " must be used and all batteries after a brief period of action stop work either through their elements becoming exhausted or by being " polarized," that is, clogged by the gases that their elements evolve. A battery that is constant has never yet been created. Furthermore a battery that would produce a current sufficiently strong to affect a small space of muscular surface for even a comparatively short time would weigh some pounds, and an " electric " belt is a thing of ounces.

Some of these belts are nothing more than bits of metal and webbing. Others are a string of discs of magnetized steel or small magnets sewn in or on some material. In the latter case the venders will gravely place a needle on the belt and call your attention to the manner in which the " electricity " attracts it. The effect of a few little magnets in contact with the human body is much about the same as that of one drop of water on a duck's back. If, however, you will insist on having an " electric " belt, buy a half dozen 5c magnets in a toy store and sew them in the band of your trousers. They will be quite as effective — or useless — as the much advertised belts for which you are asked to pay several dollars and are obviously cheaper.

These belts are much recommended by their makers for weakness of the organs of sex. Even if they could produce the results claimed for them, impotency would be produced just that much quicker, because of unnatural stimulation. There is but one proper means of building up strength of the generative powers, and that is to strengthen the entire muscular and nervous system by regular exercise.

Stop trying to get something for nothing. Leave electric belts alone, unless you are anxious to rid yourself of your money. If you want the health, strength, virility and vitality of fully developed manhood or womanhood, WORK for that superb condition. You can secure it in no other way.

# CHAPTER V

## DANGER OF STIMULATING DRUGS

### They Weaken and Destroy Through Their Reactionary Effects.

Let it be stated with all the emphasis possible that no stimulative drugs or tonics of any description, can be of the slightest service in re-creating manly virility or strengthening sexual power. The remedy must come from within, and must be the result of the building up of all the physical forces by those means which Nature has placed at our disposal in so liberal a fashion.

Stimulants of all kinds are of a harmful nature, especially those which act upon the organs of sex, either directly or indirectly. All of the advertised " remedies " for loss of vitality are of the class in question.

They affect the genital functions by causing congestion or inducing a degree of inflammation, the result in both cases being an abnormal flow of blood to the parts involved and an apparent but really disastrous revival of the activities of the organ. If a person on the verge of death was given a shock of electricity there would be a momentary spasm of false strength which would cause a heavy draft on his remaining vitality. But no one in his sober senses would claim that the muscular contortions induced by the shock were a sign of returning health. Yet the electricity was a "stimulant" nevertheless and behaved exactly as all stimulants do. That is to say, it made a demand on the meagre reserve stock of the vitality of the patient that the latter was bound to comply with. And when the temporary effects of the shock had passed the last state of the patient was worse than the first.

"In instances where debility is indicated

by a general depression of the functional duties, the use of stimulants cannot be recommended because of the reactionary effects which in many cases follow on their administration. Especially is this true where nervous, pulmonary or heart troubles exist."—*Paul G. Hendy, M.D.*

Do not be deceived. You cannot get something out of nothing. Your common sense should tell you that the one way of regaining your lost strength and virility is by going to the only source of all strength—Nature. Also should that same sense show you the folly of expecting permanent good from the stimulative compounds put up and advertised by the patent medicine impostors. Webster defines a stimulant as something that excites, rouses, urges. That's exactly it. A stimulant is the spur to the exhausted horse, the lash to the lagging mule. But notice that Webster says nothing about a stimulant being a cure or a remedy. Therein he differs from the "I-cure-men" frauds. It "rouses and urges" and because it does as much to the already worn-out victim of sexual or parental excesses, the undertakers are much more busy than they would otherwise be.

The devilish ingenuity of those who fatten on the sufferings of de-vitalized manhood is never more in evidence than in the case of these "remedies" that consist of some form of poisonous stimulant. Following the use of such comes a depression of the mental and physical powers and a corresponding craving for more of the stuff. In a short time the unhappy sufferer has formed a habit for the drug upon which the patent medicine man counts for his profits. It is not long before the victim is living, if living it may be called, upon the "remedy." Each dose makes a further demand upon his shrinking stock of vitality and with each comes a profounder reaction which calls for larger and more frequent pulls at the bottle. Finally there comes a time when the wrecked system refuses to respond to the spur and collapse ensues. But the gap in the ranks of the wretched dupes of the quack is quickly filled and the process is repeated indefinitely. It is " murder most foul and most unnatural."

Those stimulants which are especially designed to arouse the sexual organs into renewed or abnormal activity are dangerous in the extreme. Very often they defeat their purpose by causing inflammatory or other conditions which prevent the organs from fulfilling their functions. If, however, they do bring about a temporary stimulation — which is not often — such stimulation must be paid for by subsequent weakness or in some instances by permanent impotence.

The drugs which give a false hunger, which cause the kidneys to overwork themselves, which breed a spurious strength, which lend a momentary aid to a fogged brain, are all in the same category. They are bad, worse, or worst. And those who prescribe or advertise them are the enemies of humanity, and should be treated as such.

"We are a nation of drug topers. Whether this be the outcome of our temperament, of our credulity, or of the ingenuity of those whose business it is to make and advertise cure-alls I can hardly say, but the fact remains. I will not say that every one of the patented compounds before the public is of a deleterious nature, but I am quite satisfied that all of them work incalculable harm to the public health because they are taken indiscriminately and almost always continuously. The basis of not a few of them is alcohol or some other stimulant, usually of a poisonous nature, and the moral evil wrought by their use is, in consequence, of a shocking nature. Of the functional disarrangements brought about by them I will not speak except to say that every doctor in practice has among his patients not a few who are afflicted with troubles clearly traceable to the compound of a 'patent' kind."—*Jesse F. Richter, M.D.*

## CHAPTER VI

# VIRILITY SHOULD LAST AS LONG AS LIFE

### That is Nature's Intention and if Otherwise the Blame is Ours.

A popular belief which is nevertheless a fallacy, assumes that because a man is well on in years he is, or is on the eve of, becoming impotent. Now the truth is that the sexual powers, if given a moderate amount of care, should last as long as life, and a man who allows them to slip away from him has no one to blame but himself for his loss. So too can he blame no one if he allows his impotence to remain permanent.

Many men become impotent years before the advent of old age, for the simple reason that they allow the general physical health to decline, and fail to make the necessary and natural efforts to regain it, overlooking the fact that from it spring the things which give spice, enthusiasm and zest to life, including that noblest of the gifts of the Almighty — sexual virility.

That exhilaration, that excess of healthful energy, which is in evidence in the case of every vigorous man in fine physical condition, is really nothing more than a manifestation of the buoyant influence of abundant nervous or sexual strength — both really mean the same thing. Wherever you find a man possessed of the one he will always be possessed of the other to an equal degree.

Let it be restated and re-emphasized that the condition of the procreative organs is always in line with the condition of the body considered as a whole.

All loss of sexual strength is apparently accompanied by a general physical decline, but as a matter of fact the former is the outcome of the latter and not vice versa. Because of their neglect in keeping their physical forces up to a normal standard more men become partially or wholly impotent than from any other cause not even excepting excessive intercourse or other violations of the laws of sex.

No man, regardless of age, has the slightest excuse for allowing his powers, in this way, to become impaired or rendered useless. Virility should last as long as life itself. As long as one is not a bed-ridden invalid, or is not suffering from some incurable or chronic disease there is not the slightest excuse for anyone losing, temporarily or otherwise, that distinguishing mark of manhood, a robust power of sex.

If a man therefore neglects regular exercise, if no attention is given to those laws of diet and hygiene that are of such vast importance in the acquirement and retainment of vigorous health, he must expect his strength to gradually decline with the prospect of a coincident lessening of the sexual powers.

In early manhood when the vital forces are particularly strong, one may not conform to the laws of health and yet apparently possess the physical and mental vigor that is identified with superb vitality. But this will last only for a time. Premature loss of general health and sexual vigor is bound to follow and ere he reaches middle age, the victim of his own folly will be bitterly bewailing his lost or impaired manhood. Neglect yourself and just as sure as effect follows cause debility of every sort will replace your erstwhile glorious strength.

That the assertion which heads this chapter is not merely theoretical is amply proven by the returns of the departments of vital statistics of many big centres of population. Apart from that, we have some notable illustrations of the permanence of the vital powers under favorable conditions in the persons of notable public men.

But the prevention of premature impotence can be readily accomplished, and sexual powers that have apparently gone for ever can be revived in their entirety.

We can promise a recovery and a strengthening of these powers with a certainty, absolute and unfailing, provided that the sufferer accurately and regularly follows the rules we have laid down in this work for strengthening the nervous organism, so bringing about a renaissance of physical vigor and thus resurrecting from the grave of weakness those gifts, the possession of which gives a man the three dearest things of life — home, wife, children.

## CHAPTER VII

## MAGNIFICENT MANHOOD

### Foundation Upon which Rests Everything in Life.

Superb manhood is the foundation of the race and all that appertains to it. Through it man shares with the Almighty that most wonderful and comprehensive of all powers — the power of giving life to a mass of lifeless atoms. According to Scripture the first ancestor of all, Adam, was shaped of clay and then there was breathed into the inanimate form the "breath of life" and forthwith it saw, felt, heard and moved. Eve was also the outcome of a Divine miracle, but after that, the task of creating other human lives was delegated to man. "Increase and multiply," was the command and with it came those sexual gifts that made its fulfilment possible. Nor was the order issued to man alone. Organized beings from the highest to the lowest heard it, were equipped for it, and obeyed it.

"The principle of sex continues from the highest organized form down to the minutest animalculæ. In no animal is the reproductive apparatus less simple than it is in the higher plants; that is to say, in every instance there are two organs — a germ-preparing and a germ-nourishing. These organs differ in form and complexity of structure but their essential function is the same after all."— *Dr. A. Carpenter, in Principles of Human Physiology.*

Primeval man was probably the possessor of perfect sexual powers and the nervous and muscular strength that goes with them. Our fellow beings, that we are pleased to call the lower animals, have retained such powers in all their original vigor. But we, or at least a great many of us, have failed to guard the sacred trust reposed in us. The errors of parents, our own unbridled passions, neglect of our bodies and artificial modes of life have all done their part in robbing us of the most precious of the many gifts of nature. We are in too many cases destitute of that which alone brings satisfying happiness to ourselves, and to coming generations—robust sexuality allied to the noble qualities which follow in its wake.

Think of the marvel and mystery of the conception of life. There is a commingling of bodies and that which a few moments before was, as the chemist would declare, a group of inorganic elements—molecules of carbon, hydrogen, oxygen, silicon, calcium and nitrogen—is impregnated with a force, or condition that results in their "living." Just what this living or life is, is a profound problem that has defied the speculations and investigations of sages and savants, theologians and philosophers since man began to theorize on his origin, and ponder on his future, and this wonderful secret of life may never become known to human minds.

The gift of life includes all other gifts. The crowned monarch sits upon his throne. He either has or can command everything that existence yields, with perhaps the exception of health. The arts and sciences pay him tribute, his armies and fleets guarantee him glory, his people render loyal obedience, his counsellors guide his feet in the ways of safety on earth, and his prelates smooth his path to the Hereafter. Life to him is charged to the brim with the things that make life worth living.

Then comes the crack of the assassin's revolver, and out of a tiny hole oozes that mystic, elusive yet tremendously real thing, that we call life. And now what are power and glory and riches to the dead man and what is he to them? Nothing! Life has gone and with its going all else has gone also. Given life and all things are possible, take it away and what can be accomplished? Life is everything, for lacking it, there is nothing. It is the tangible manifestation of the Something that keeps the wheels of the universe in operation.

If men then would reflect on the tremendous responsibilities and possibilities that centre around their faculty of giving life to atoms of otherwise dead matter, in other words of reproducing their kind, they would value that power above all else and shrink with horror from any act which might tend to weaken or destroy it. Yet how few of us realize the sacredness of the sexual function or understand the immutable intimacy between it and all the other phases or aspects of man's existence.

It can be laid down as a principle from which there is never a departure that Nature amply rewards a man who sees the importance of conserving his sexual energies, and employs proper methods to that end. She crowns him with mag-

nificent health, she endows him with that irresistible quality which, for want of a better name, we call animal magnetism, she makes him successful socially, professionally and — most of all — in the home circle. The unswerving law of the survival of the fittest is at work in his behalf and is doing its best to make him fit and yet more fit to survive — in the persons of his children. He tingles to the finger tips with the nervous energy that is the accompaniment of perfect sexuality. He is an emphatic proof of the fact that he whose life is rounded out on lines of true manhood must as a natural necessity, be possessed of the first essential to such manhood, sexual virility.

Such virility is in truth the mainspring of human action. It is not only the fountain but the foundation of lives, and lives of the purest, the strongest and the most useful at that.

The fiery ardor of a patriot, the devotion of a religious enthusiast, the inspiration to noble deeds of valor, the sacrificial, patriotic spirit that has time and again caused the world to ring with praises of some hero, all spring from the basic nervous energy which supplies the power of sex, the force of perfected manhood.

Name any man famous in the worlds of literature, of art, or of science, and in nearly every instance he will be found to possess evidences of strong virility. The intense energy, so necessary to the labor which has brought him success, is the same that controls and vitalizes his sexual gifts.

"Sexuality has been strongly marked in all the great men who have risen to eminence in all departments of life; without it man would be mean, selfish, sordid and ungracious to his fellowmen and uncivil to womankind. Were it not for this nature which God has implanted in our being, no man would desire to provide for the support of another individual, or enter into a relation which would be likely to impose upon him the necessity of supporting a family of dependent and growing children. No man becomes affable, gracious and considerate to women until he is rendered so by the awakening of his sexual nature and the quickening of that within him, which, when held under proper discipline and control, renders him noble and unselfish."—*Sylvanus Stall, D.D.*

The importance of strong sexuality cannot be too strongly emphasized. Its influence on life is marvelous. If a vigorous man acquires a complaint or gets into a condition that weakens his sexual organs, his powers in every way will begin to suffer — his muscles will grow flabby, his nerves will be affected, and unless a change is quickly made, he will soon become a physical wreck without hope, ambition or desire. The nervous, sexual, muscular and vital forces are so closely interwoven that what affects one for evil always influences the others in a similar manner.

But per contra as steps are taken to recover lost strength and vitality in the way that this book relates, as the muscles are developed and hardened, as the whole system is " tuned up " there is a return of the nervous powers in general and the sexuality of the man once more asserts itself.

Splendid sexuality never makes its fortunate possessor a sensualist any more than does great muscular strength make its owner a thug or bully. On the contrary those who are blessed with superb manhood are usually faithful lovers and devoted husbands. It is such men that are the hope of the race in the future as they are its ornaments in the present; for theirs it is to set their weaker brethren examples of what they too may be, and transmit their physical and moral virtues to posterity. And such men invariably marry, for with the wisdom that comes from their clear, forceful mentalities they know that it is not well for man to be alone, and that the life perfect is one that is shared with another.

"A true and permanent union of one man to one woman establishes a relation of affection and interests which can in no other way be made to exist between two human beings. Without such an union no individual can be considered as having answered the whole purpose of his existence, or as having arrived at the full development of which his character is capable. He is incomplete and imperfect. He has tendencies, and capacities and powers for good which have never been called into activity and which he may not even know exist. Domestic life and the domestic relation are the essential elements of human happiness and human progress so far as moral and spiritual characteristics are concerned. From this same source — domesticity — proceeds our purest happiness and upon it depends our highest motives, those that tend to goodness and improvement. From the relations of the sexes spring all that gives charm, grace and true value to human intercourse. Without it there would be no families, no relatives; none of those thousand endearing associations which arise from them. Strike out from the life of man all the hopes, interests and motives which grow out of this relation and what would be left him but a desolate and merely brutal existence."—*John Ware, M.D.*

# CHAPTER VIII

## LOSS OF MANLY POWERS

### Causes of Weakness, Debility and Partial or Entire Impotence.

Why is the man of indifferent physique and weakened or defunct sexual powers so common, and why is he of superb health and vitality so relatively rare? Let me try to tell you.

Nature is in some respects the sternest of teachers. She has no patience with, no pity for the ignorant. Deliberate violations of her laws on the part of the perverse are severely punished, but none the less is he chastised who is a law-breaker through lack of knowledge. Man, the king of all animals, as a race, still grovels in the dust and mire of ignorance, and even his boasted knowledge sometimes turns on him to sting and not infrequently destroy him. Such knowledge is too often a knowledge of evil without a corresponding realization of its effects and certainly none of its antidotes. This combination of harmful wisdom and more harmful ignorance it is that is responsible for the millions of sexual and physical wrecks that are strewing the shores of our civilizations in ever increasing numbers.

They have knowledge of the momentary pleasures which can be obtained from sexual indulgences, without the knowledge of their terribly deleterious influence under certain conditions. Knowledge of but one half the meaning of the word sexuality and ignorance of the other half. Truly a little knowledge is a dangerous thing and never more so than in matters relating to the questions of manhood. Let the emasculated creatures that once were high spirited boys or hopeful young men whom one meets in our schools on our streets point the moral in this connection. Ask them if they would be that which they are if the prudishness of parents or the mock modesty of public opinion had not prevented them from learning that they have learned all too late. And their reply in spirit if not in letter will be "If we only had known, if we only had known!"

To repeat, ignorance of facts having to do with the sexual instinct and functions that should be as plain as the noonday sun to every human being, together with a stupid disregard of the laws of health so necessary to build up a vigorous and symmetrical body, have resulted in the filling of civilized countries with a host of pigmies and weaklings.

The chief cause of premature loss of manly vitality is unquestionably masturbation or self abuse. And the predisposition to masturbation is almost always that mischievous secrecy maintained on sexual subjects by those whose solemn duty it is to instruct, to warn and to watch the children committed to their care. And so the boy, with the natural curiosity of budding youth being unable to gratify it elsewhere, turns to his older and more "knowing" companions with the result that he is forthwith initiated into the frightful mysteries of the vice. Or he may even discover it by accident and not knowing its powers for evil indulge in it constantly until his vitality gives up the struggle for mastery finding that it has an enemy with which it literally has no chance. If a boy finally escapes from the clutches of this Gorgon evil—though many never do—he finds that he is afflicted with night losses that seem to waste his vitality almost as thoroughly as did the vice whose grip he has just broken.

Or there may be involuntary drains upon his vitality during the day, or the general lowering of his physical and mental states due to his past excesses may further weaken him. Then there are a half hundred other possible bodily complications that arise from and still further speed his lessening manhood toward the goal of impotency.

"The evils resulting from a violation of nature's method of growth by a life of early dissipation are physical, mental and moral. In some organizations the former, in some the latter are observable in the most marked degree, but no one can escape either the physical deterioration or the mental degradation which results from the irrational and un-human exercise of the great endowment of sex."—*Mark J. Boody, M.D.*

If he escapes with approximately good health, however, he is fairly sure to practice promiscuous intercourse with fallen women. It will not be long before he pays the penalty of his sin and folly. Sooner or later he will be made to realize that Nature, through the medium of the most frightful diseases known to humanity, has placed the seal of her displeasure on acts that drag a man down to — no, lower than, the lowest beast.

Then indeed are the torture of his body and mind of a terrible nature. Visions of complete loss of manhood confront him. He may have had dreams of a home, a loving wife, and happy, beautiful children. He realizes that the disease from which he is suffering may forever destroy the possibility of the realization of this hope, and he will curse the day when the harlot came into his life to wrack his body with agony, to charge his bones with corruption and to destroy in him the one thing that makes a man.

Should he pass through the ordeal with enough remaining vitality and sexual appetite to decide on getting married, the girl who can be induced to accept him is usually of weak temperament and void of that normal instinct of her sex which prompts her to draw the line between legitimate intercourse and sensual excess. And again indignant Nature intervenes to the end of depriving the man of the gift which he so brutally misuses and the woman of health and happiness.

There are many other causes of loss of manhood, some of which begin at birth when the victims are encumbered with clothing that prevents rather than encourages muscular movements. Then they are compelled to breathe foul air when the weather is cold; they are always overfed; the bottle often does duty for the mother's breast, and they come in contact with all sorts of conditions that tend to steal from them their vitality. Of course over half the children subject to this treatment are killed by it, while those that survive never attain the superb manhood that is their inalienable right.

And so this is our civilization as applied to that most important of all the questions that affect humanity — how to insure and maintain the manhood of our race. Yet what do we find?

First the baby so dressed and used and fed that the deterioration of its incipient powers of manhood is begun forthwith.

Next the youthful victim of masturbation, he being so because of the damnable neglect of parents to warn their children of this evil which degrades and demoralizes their physical and sexual systems and makes all the vices that attend it so easily acquired.

Following is the young man, the patron of the social evil whose "weakness" is winked at by society and whose lusts are ministered to by a horde of panderers.

Lastly there is the married libertine who continues in the marriage the unbridled license of his bachelor days.

And finally is the decrepit, tottering skeleton, once a man, only arrived at middle age and a monument to the "civilized" conditions that have made him what he is.

I speak knowingly and from my heart-core when I declare that as long as such a state of affairs exists, we have no more right to the claim of civilization and advancement than had those effeminate, corrupt and well-fed patricians of ancient Rome whose weakness, moral and physical, resulted in the downfall of that great empire.

The decay and death of not only Rome but of other past civilizations of the Old World convey a lesson that can not be mistaken, and the writer insists with all possible emphasis that either existing conditions will soon have to be changed or else the country and all that appertains to it in the way of power and prestige of which we boast will encounter swift oblivion.

Think you there is no truth in this statement? Let the future answer!

But **cry** out your beliefs on the housetops!

## CHAPTER IX

# RAVAGES OF MASTURBATION

### It is the Parent of Misery, Emasculation and Insanity.

It is an amazing fact that the parent who is most solicitous for the spiritual well being of a son, who makes every effort, and, if need be, sacrifice, to insure him an educational training of the best, who is careful of his health, who is anxious in regard to his companions, who, in short has the moral, mental and physical welfare of the child profoundly at heart, will nevertheless neglect to enlighten and instruct him on the most vital issue of his existence, his sexuality and what is involved in its use and abuse. His education on this point is left to others and with what disastrous results, let the hospitals, the wrecked homes and the insane asylums proclaim.

It is a terrible charge to make, but the fact remains that the prevalance of that most insiduous of vices, masturbation, must be laid at the door of the unwisely silent parent. The laws of sex should be as plain as the alphabet to every human being, even from early childhood, yet boys grow up without a word being said to them on this important subject. They come in contact with the most destructive evil of life, self-abuse, before the real struggle of life begins. They enter languid and enervated because of the want of a preliminary word of warning.

Think of it, reader. Parents who claim to love their children, allow this.

" Masturbation outrages nature's sexual ordinances more than any or all the other forms of sexual sin man can perpetrate and inflicts consequences the most terrible. It is man's sin of sins, and vice of vices; and has caused incomparably more sexual dilapidation, paralysis, and disease, as well as demoralization, than all the other sexual depravities combined. Neither Christendom nor heathendom suffers any evil at all to compare with this; because of its universality, and its terribly fatal ravages on body and mind; and because it attacks the young idols of our hearts, and hopes of our future years. Pile all other evils together — drunkenness upon all cheateries, swindlings, robberies, and murders; and tobacco upon both, for it is the greatest scourge; and all sickness, diseases and pestilences upon all; and war as the cap sheaf of them all — and all combined cause not a tithe as much human deterioration and misery as does this secret sin."— *Prof. O. S. Fowler.*

You, reader, must have had cases of the effects of the vice come under your observation ere now. You have seen a strong, handsome boy, clear-eyed with beautifully-tinted complexion, straight, well-formed limbs. You have admired his elastic step, his manly carriage, his symmetrically-formed body and his well-poised head denoting character, courage, self-reliance and manliness.

A year, or even a few months, intervene, and this boy has in the interval learned this secret vice. You see him again, and you may well start with pain and surprise at the change.

There is no light of health in his eyes now; there is no symmetry in his ungainly body, no tint to his sallow cheeks, no grace, or manliness in his bearing. He looks old and weak, appears bashful and timid, and afraid of your glance. The dark circles under his eyes, unshapely appearance of his lower limbs, and generally decrepit and demoralized condition tell a tale that no language can fittingly render; he is a wretched devotee of masturbation.

"The most fruitful source of self-pollution is ignorance. If parents were faithful in the discharge of their duty to their children in this respect, the evil would be generally corrected. The silence of most parents is both foolish and culpable. The person who leaves his or her child to learn from vicious companions in an unhallowed way what they should have received from the lips of father or mother is guilty of grave neglect, and loses the best opportunity of a parent's life to establish the mind of the child in purity and virtue."—*Sylvanus Stall, D. D.*

Mrs. Alice Lee Moque, herself the mother of three boys, in writing upon this subject correctly and pathetically says:

"Ignorance is a dreadful sin. In this enlightened age we must recognize that ignorance is not innocence, and remember that to forewarn our boys is to forearm them. The truth, properly told, has never yet harmed a child; silence, false shame and mystery have corrupted the souls and bodies of untold millions."

"Rendered childless by my husband's ignorance of these private truths you teach,

I adopted three sons, whom I determined, by forewarning, to save from this vice, and warned my eldest on his sixteenth birthday, but was too late, as he owned he had perpetrated it for years. Determined to be in ample season with my other two, I warned my next youngest at thirteen, never dreaming that it could be practiced before puberty; but found myself again too late. Half frantic with disappointment, and determined to make sure of saving my now only undefiled, I warned him at ten; but, horrible to relate was still too late; for he had already learned and perpetrated it!"

Another authority on the subject gives testimony thus:

"The sin of self-pollution is one of the most destructive evils ever practiced by fallen man. In many respects it is several degrees worse than common whoredom, and leaves in its train more awful consequences. It excites the powers of nature to undue action, and produces violent secretions, which necessarily and speedily exhaust the vital principle and energy; hence the muscles become flaccid and feeble, the tone and natural action of the nerves relaxed and impeded, the understanding confused, the memory oblivious, the judgment perverted, the will indeterminate and wholly without energy to resist; the eyes appear languishing and without expression, and the countenance vacant; appetite ceases, for the stomach is incapable of performing its proper office; nutrition fails; tremors, fears, and terrors are generated; and thus the wretched victim drags out a miserable existence, till, superannuated, even before he had time to arrive at man's estate, with a mind often debilitated even to a state of idiotism, his worthless body tumbles into the grave, and his guilty soul (guilty of self-murder) is hurried into the awful presence of its Judge!"—*Adam Clarke's Com. on Onan.*

The testimony of a well known physician is to this effect:

"These results of masturbation I have seen in my own practice — involuntary emissions, prostration of strength, paralysis of the limbs, hysteria, epilepsy, strange nervous affections, dyspepsia, hypochondria, spinal disease, pain and weakness in the back and limbs, costiveness, and, in fine, the long and dismal array of gastric, enteric, nervous and spinal affections, which are so complicated and difficult to manage."—*Dr. J. A. Brown.*

And testimony on similar lines might be quoted indefinitely.

I ask those who are responsible to the Being who gave them little children what are they doing to save those children from the Hades of masturbation? What would you think of a man who would stand unmoved by a blind child and see it walk to the brink of a precipice and fall into the depth below? But where is the difference between such an inhuman creature and a parent or guardian who will carelessly watch his own little one, falling into the abyss of masturbation, which, though it may not mean death, in every case means that the victim will be somehow or in some way maimed for life? Of course he often recovers and becomes a good and useful citizen, but he would have been better and stronger and nobler if not tainted and wrecked by the influences of the vice.

There is no name too harsh to be applied to such unfeeling, prudish parents. The lowest animals protect their own progeny from destructive influences, but these so-called parents who are travesties on the name, allow their children to be ensnared in the pitfalls of this frightful vice without an attempt to give them warning, without an effort to save them, without a word of expostulation or protest.

In the name of decency, of humanity, of common kindness I bid you, parents and guardians and teachers, if you have one atom of truth, of honor, of love in your hearts, warn your *boys* — and your girls, too — of the frightful evil in question so that they may learn to hate and shun it.

Neglect this imperative duty, and if there is *Hell* in the other world, you fully deserve to learn of its existence, for you have assisted in no small way in making a hell on this earth for your own child.

*There is no crime more dastardly,* that deserves more punishment, than this miserable silence on matters about which it is absolutely essential that the child should be properly informed. Children depend on their parents for protection, and when the moral protection under consideration is denied them they would be far better off dead rather than undergoing the living death that follows on the practice of secret sensuality.

"Private fornication causes twenty times more misery than any other sexual sin. And this is substantially the opinion of all who have examined this subject. If a loved child must practice either—O merciful God! deliver all from such a dilemma—almost as soon let it DIE. Any other cup of bitterness is less bitter! Nothing, O fond parent, can render your beloved offspring more completely wretched."—*Prof. O. S. Fowler.*

Prostitution and intemperance may do much to demoralize and destroy the character and physique of young men, but unquestionably, masturbation causes more physical deterioration, more insanity, more tendency to crime, than any other one sexual form of evil. It attacks boys when they are maturing, when the mind and body are alike in their most receptive conditions, when influences brought to bear on them leave their impress through life and it vulgarizes, degrades and ruins them physically, mentally and sexually.

"Many of the ills which come upon the

young at and after puberty arise from this habit, persisted in so as to waste their vital energies, and enervate their physical and mental powers. Nature designs that this drain should be reserved until mature age, and even then be made but sparingly. Sturdy manhood, in all its vigor, loses its energy, and bends under the too frequent expenditure of this important secretion; and no age or condition will protect a man from the danger of unlimited indulgence, though legally and naturally exercised.

"In the young, however, its influence is much more seriously felt; and even those who have indulged so cautiously as not to break down their health or minds, cannot know how much their physical energy, mental vigor, and moral purity have been weakened by this indulgence. No cause produces as much insanity. The records of the institutions give an appalling catalogue of cases attributed to it."—*Dr. Woodward.*

Again and again has the question been asked, " Can the effect of this terrible evil be eradicated? " The truth is that a boy can never be the man that he might have been had he not practiced the habit, though he can undoubtedly recover from its results to the extent of developing a fine vigorous physique provided that proper efforts are made to that end. To such an unfortunate the writer would say: Take all sorts of outdoor exercises. Live in the open air as much as you can, and vow with an unflinching determination that you will be a man — that you will conquer the degrading habit that has robbed you of so much.

Remember that your will and mentality can be of the utmost service to you in assisting you to attain a speedy and complete recovery. If the vile habit still holds you in its tentacles you must determine to acquire sufficient moral strength to conquer it. YOU MUST BECOME MASTER OF

YOURSELF. This can not be accomplished at once in many cases. It takes time to work out such a revolution in your life. But you must not lose heart if you meet with failure at first, and while trying, failing or succeeding, you should be building up your physical and nervous powers. As you increase in strength and health, as you become more normal in general, you will find yourself gradually, but none the less surely, acquiring the power to overcome this evil thing. And with the aid of determination and perseverance victory is bound to be yours in the long run.

DON'T LIVE TOO MUCH BY OR WITHIN YOURSELF. Go out into the world and associate with others. Seek all sorts and all kinds of temperate and natural enjoyment. Avoid as you would the Devil himself every thought relating to sex. Let your mind be virgin as nearly as possible.

If you are unlucky enough to have nothing to do then it is your duty to find something to employ your head and hands immediately. Hard work and plenty of it is the best possible remedy for the vice in question. Your mind and your muscle should be continually busy. Labor that sends you to bed at the close of the day thoroughly fatigued, and ready and willing to fall asleep the moment your head touches the pillow, is one of the most efficient means of aiding you to break the grasp of the habit.

Results of importance cannot be achieved in a day or a week. In some instances it takes months and in some extremely bad cases, years to effect a cure, but self mastery must be sought continually and sooner or later it is certain to be yours. Learn to control yourself and your thoughts. Cultivate a love for all that is morally beautiful, for temperance of act and thought, for normality in all things. Shun evil of every sort.

If, although you have conquered the habit, you are still suffering from its effects, you must not lose hope. You must not think that you are lost physically beyond recall. Let me assure you that you can make a new man of yourself if you only determine to do so. You can build for yourself a new body and new nerves. You can develop renewed muscular power and nervous power. You become again a man if, patiently and day after day you work faithfully for the rich rewards that go with the attainment of superb manhood.

Let the dead past bury the dead. You have a new life that is to be lived in the present and in the future. Dedicate this life to all that is noble, good and true. Cast out all thoughts relative to the erotic delusions of the life behind you. Think of the joy of life and health that is certainly in store for you in the future. And vow that you will accomplish that which will insure your becoming a magnificent man, that will give you the enviable powers of a perfect man.

Of course, the writer admits that one of the lamentable outcomes of the habit of masturbation is a loss of vitality which can never be fully replaced no matter how sincere and patient are the efforts of he who is striving for physical and moral redemption. In other words the ex-masturbator cannot become the perfect specimen of manhood that he might have been had he never sinned. But he or you, my friend, if you too have cause to regret an acquaintance with the vice, can unquestionably acquire that which may be termed normal power. You may by means about to be related secure good health, good spirits and fair sexual ability. So do not permit yourself to unduly suffer from the pangs of useless remorse. A morbid habit of thought is not infrequently a result of the vice. Remember this when you are tempted to believe that you have sinned beyond pardon or have injured yourself physically beyond all means of cure. Such gloomy beliefs exist in your imagination only and not in the domain of fact. Once for all let it be said with due emphasis that you can again become a MAN if you are willing to make every effort to bring about that most desirable result.

For those who are still in the clutch of this mighty evil, and are striving to regain their freedom, I would suggest that a daily régime be adopted such as follows:

Upon awakening in the morning jump out of bed on the instant and go through some vigorous exercise which will bring into play all the muscles of the body. The exercises given in chapter XXXII for building vital power can be recommended for this purpose. Follow, with a cold bath, using a wet towel or wet sponge, after which thoroughly dry the body with a rough towel.

Don't wear too heavy clothing. Wear

just as few garments as will enable you to keep moderately warm. Let the air come in free contact with the body. If you can take air baths at frequent opportunities, either in your room or out of doors, do so. They are of the utmost value.

Remember to oust from your mind all thoughts of a sexually depraved nature. Confine your diet to two meals per day, drinking freely of water between meals. If you have no desire for at least a glass of water every two or three hours, you should try to form the habit of taking such. If you have no wholesome occupation find one at the earliest opportunity. If you are not doing manual work some time during the day you should take a long walk. But in any event keep yourself busy.

Eat your first meal at twelve or one o'clock. Masticate every morsel of food very thoroughly before swallowing. Eat your second meal about six hours after your first meal and three or four hours before retiring.

Keep the windows of your sleeping room wide open. The purer the atmosphere of your room the better it will be for you. Cover yourself in bed as lightly as possible and yet be able to retain warmth. Don't retire for the night until you are sufficiently fatigued to go to sleep immediately. Don't loll in bed under any conditions. If you find that you are not sleepy get up and walk around, or take some light exercise until you feel that your eyes are getting heavy with need of slumber.

# CHAPTER X

## EVILS OF PROMISCUOUS INTERCOURSE

This Vice Makes Physical Wrecks and Moral Derelicts by the Thousands.

Sexual intercourse of an illegitimate nature is, like all other forms of law-breaking, the fosterer of much evil. The basis of physical intimacy between the sexes should be sincere affection rooted in mutual respect and regard. Any other kind of passion is bestial and even unnatural and in not a few cases is as productive of physical and mental harm as is masturbation itself.

A young man in order to gratify his desires for promiscuous intercourse must either rob an innocent girl of her virtue, consort with unchaste women in private life or seek the society of prostitutes. In the first instance he commits a dastardly crime; in the second he risks reputation at the least; and in the third, he takes chances of so frightful a sort that did he but reflect upon them he would turn with shuddering disgust from the purchased embraces of his companion.

And yet, such is the fatuity of a man intoxicated and debased by lust, that in nine cases out of ten he hunts for a "Scarlet Woman" when under its influence. In doing so he is exchanging the maximum of risks for the minimum of enjoyment. For reciprocity of mind and body is necessary to the true understanding of the sexual relation, so that he gets scant pleasure from one who is assuredly indifferent to him and who endures his society only for what she gains by it in a financial way.

This would be bad enough anyhow, for where there is no mutuality of feeling, one or the other gives up a large amount of nervous vitality. In the case of a congenial union this vitality is returned and not lost to its original possessor. This it is that makes the ideal marriage a source of such deep pleasure without entailing on the partners to it, drains on their energies.

But this loss of nervous force is the least of the ills which wait on he who cohabits with courtesans. Nature has set a price upon fornication that none can afford to give. She takes her pay in nervous power, and physical health. No man who makes a habit of visiting these women ever escapes the penalties of so doing for long, and these take the aspect of diseases of the most loathsome character. Go to any of the hospitals and see the myriads of sufferers from horrifying ailments that at times eat the flesh from the body, leaving great open sores that are healed only by death, or cause literal rotting of the bones, or destroy the tissues of the throat and the substance of the gums, denude the patient's head of hair, gnaw away his features, cause him to be a fœtid mass of constant agony and then ponder on the rewards that wait on promiscuous intercourse.

"Promiscuous intercourse leads to gonorrhœa, gleet, syphilis, stricture, diseased offspring, childlessness, and many other evils. Almost the entire civilized race is to-day tainted with venereal poison. If we imagine vitality divided into equal portions, each item may be looked upon as canceled by an act of cohabitation. Then it is obvious that the more frequent these acts of intercourse, the sooner the stock of vital power must be exhausted."—*A. F. Reinhold, Ph.D., M.D.*

As in the case of masturbation no small proportion of the youthful victims of venereal diseases, are such because of the asinine prudishness which observes in the family circle. That the task of talking to a son about the dangers that threaten his blossoming manhood is as delicate as it is difficult, is admitted. But not a few duties are difficult. What parent or relative would shrink from the discharge of this one thought after reading the following vivid picture of the aftermath of intercourse with loose women:

"God in nature condemns sexual depravities as the most utterly abominable in His holy sight of all others, and affixes to them the seal of His uttermost reprobation, by appending to them pains and penalties more painful, and loathsomeness more disgusting than to any other sins and vices. Natural expression always tells the truth, and nothing but the truth, though by no means the whole truth here, for that is impossible, even by this Heaven's most eloquent orator. A strong man or woman slowly atoning, by lingering, agonizing moments, hours, days and months, till a protracted death finally closes upon the scene, the author never has seen, never desires to see. Other pens, more vivid, have attempted this painful description, only confessedly to fall far short of its awful realities. What feverish days! What restless nights! What agonizing aches and pains in every bone, and muscle, and nerve! What eyes rolling and glaring and protruding, as if internal agonies were pushing them out of their sockets! An awful stench nauseates beyond any power of description. A putrid human carcass — beast does not, cannot suffer this — is livid with poison! Running sores here, there, everywhere, ejecting excretions how utterly disgusting!"—*Prof O. S. Fowler.*

The description of the suffering of the youthful dissolute are, as its author suggests, under rather than overdrawn. The "lock-ward" of a public hospital is as near an approach to the Hades of popular fancy and tradition as one can well imagine. Insulted nature seems to have expended herself in devising terrifically agonizing punishments for this sort of moral and physical weakling who represents a disgusted miscarriage of her plans.

"If men whose abnormal desires lead them into the ways of promiscuous intercourse could but see some one or more of the victims to be found at all times in any of the large hospitals — the foul, loathsome ulcer; the poison eating away gradually, slowly, but surely, the flesh; the eyes gone, the nose destroyed, giving the face a most hideous aspect; the bones of the skull eaten, exposing the brain; the mark of manhood obliterated altogether, a loathsome, living death — they would think twice before venturing into the meshes of her whose 'feet take hold on hell.' The breaking of no human law entails on the wrong-doer such fearfully prompt, repulsive and incurable penalties as does the unnatural one of miscellaneous intercourse. The very first transgression ofttimes develops the poison of syphilis, the non-desire for which may be inferred from what one of the most distinguished of French surgeons has said: ' I would not have a chancre of the size of a pin's head on my person for all Paris.' "—*John Cowan, M.D.*

But not syphilis alone is the cause of lasting pain and more or less premature death. Gonorrhœa, usually spoken of by the man-about-town, as " not a bit worse than a cold," leaves behind it even after an apparent cure, a host of evils, some dangerous, others less so, but all conspiring to rob the victim of energy and strength. Ask the man who suffers from a stricture following a " cured " case of gonorrhœa what he thinks of the latter disease and between groans of blood-sweating agony he will tell you that he is enduring the tortures of the damned. Or those afflicted with incurable gleet, or bladder affections or recurrent attacks of iritis, or chronic weakness and inflammations of some parts of the organs of sex — put the same question to them and note the answers that they will give to you.

How many physically perfect men, some of them athletes, has not the writer seen reduced to ghastly wrecks by some one of these diseases? How many lives once filled with promise has he not seen charged with hopeless suffering by them. How many prospective good citizens, happy husbands and affectionate fathers has he not noted who were transformed into miserable nonentities by them. And still the diabolical work goes on. The demand for diseased courtesans is actually created by a diseased prudery, and to finish it all, the only possible means of curing the sufferers are ignored or neglected by the medical profession.

Any of these diseases are accompanied by a serious loss of sexual strength, but this is not only on account of the general physical decline that accompanies and follows them, but is due to the fact that the ordinary curative treatment is often extremely harsh, and the strong drugs, ejections, etc., that are used, leave traces of their weakening influences years after they have been discontinued in the shape of nervous or organic disorders brought into being by them.

Regardless of what opinion may be held as to the desirability of absolute continence, no reasoning process can possibly cause a man to conclude that promiscuous intercourse is either beneficial or desirable. This, even if one is laboring under the delusion that he is too careful to acquire any of the terrible maladies that are the penalties for infractions of nature's plain sexual laws.

" Among the passions of the future man which at this period (youth) should be strictly restrained, is that of physical love or lust, for none wars so completely against the principles which have been laid down as the most conducive to long and useful lives. No other excess so thoroughly lessens the sum of the vital powers, none so much weakens the vital organs, none is more active in hastening the dissolution of all the vital faculties and none so totally prohibits restoration. I could if I would, draw a frightful picture of the results of these passionate excesses."—*Erasmus Wilson, the famous British surgeon.*

Of the side issues of promiscuous intercourse nothing has been said so far. But ask a police court magistrate what in his opinion is the main cause of young men becoming thieves, drunkards, gamblers, forgers, or murderers, and he will unhesitatingly reply: "Fast women."

"Many of your patients will ask you about sexual intercourse and expect you to prescribe fornication. I would just as soon prescribe theft or lying or anything else that God has forbidden. Continence does no harm to mind or body, its discipline is excellent, marriage can be safely waited for and among the many nervous and hypochondriacal patients who have talked to me about fornication I have never heard one say that he was better or happier for it."—*Sir James Page, M.D., Chemical Lectures.*

# CHAPTER XI

## SPERMATORRHEA

Mysterious Drains Upon Nervous Powers — The Life Fluid Often Oozes Away Unperceived — These Drains Lessen Vital Power and Should be Remedied.

Apart from the drains upon the sexual powers which have been recited in this volume, there are others of so insiduous a nature that the victim of them is hardly conscious of their existence. It is only when his attention is called to the fact that his linen is slightly but persistently moistened, or that the aperture of his sexual organ is usually damp, that he begins to suspect that all is not well with him, and that he is losing more or less constantly that vital fluid which is life itself — the semen.

But in most cases he is not cognizant of the fact that his vitality and sexual force are being stealthily, but none the less surely, sapped in the manner described. He only knows that he is nervous, irritable and debilitated, that his digestion is indifferent, his sleep broken and feverish, his days full of depression and forebodings, that he has lost all relish for the healthy and wholesome things of life, that a little exertion, mental or physical, causes him to feel "played out" and that he acts and looks like an old man before he is a properly developed young one.

Possibly he may, through his unaided efforts, try to regain his lost buoyancy of spirits and physical vigor. Or he may fall into the hands of quacks, in which case he is to be pitied indeed, for it is the policy of these fellows to prolong rather than to alleviate or cure his trouble. Or, again, he may consult a physician in good standing who will in nine cases out of ten make a diagnosis of an honest but mistaken nature. And in the meantime the seminal fluid is oozing from him in minute but never ceasing quantities. His life is literally going out from him and he knows it not. The ensuing breakdown of his system may be deferred for years, but it is inevitable, nevertheless, unless the trouble is detected in time and steps are taken to check its powers for evil. This form of spermatorrhea is all the more dangerous because it does its work in so undemonstrative a fashion.

Weakness of the glands, muscles and nerves of the sexual apparatus is directly responsible for this malady and such a condition is generally the outcome of a lowerering of the tone of the system by masturbation, and other errors of youth. Sexual excesses, in or out of wedlock, will also induce it by causing debility of the body as a whole and the organs of generation in particular. To use a homely simile, the trouble may be compared to a leaky faucet, the metal work or washer of which being worn and weakened by excessive use, allows of a constant dripping of water.

A demonstration of the trouble can be brought about in a number of ways. If the victim talks to, sits near or caresses a woman, a clear viscid fluid will ooze from the opening of the penis, which does not resemble semen very much, but which it is nevertheless, or, to speak with accuracy, it is semen mixed with mucus. The same kind of thing takes place under the influence of lewd books, pictures or conversation, unduly tight clothing, bicycle or horseback riding, retention of urine, too many coverings in bed, alcoholic drinks, and in some cases, excitement of any kind whatever.

Constipation, and consequent straining at stool, is responsible for a larger and more apparent loss than any of the other causes recited. This is because the muscular exertion required involves the weakened sexual apparatus. In some instances the mingled semen and mucus will issue from the penis in an unbroken stream during the efforts made to evacuate the bowels. It need hardly be added that additional weakness and losses are the outcome of such exertions so that if you are constipated, adopt those methods that will quickly bring you relief. If you cannot readily obtain foods that will effect a satisfactory cure, use the internal flushing treatment spoken of elsewhere until you find an effective relaxing diet. Remember, also, never to strain while the male organ is congested with blood. If it is absolutely necessary for you to strain to have a passage press the fingers on the outside of the urethra just under the scrotum while straining and be sure that the organ is relaxed, for then there is far less danger of a loss of semen.

There are a good many physicians who, if they discover a trouble of the kind in question, will prescribe tonics or some other drugs. Such are useless and worse than useless. Tear up the prescriptions and realize that there is but one way of curing cases of this description and that is by using natural methods of regaining and increasing the muscular, nervous and functional powers. Powders, potions and pills are alike valueless.

If you are guilty of sexual excesses, you must immediately cease them. If you are conscious of other evil in your life, eliminate it.

A régime such as is recommended in this book will be effective, provided you coincidentally live a pure life. Increased nervous power will remedy your trouble, and this can only be obtained by following a strict series of rules for improving your general physical condition.

The exercises in Chapter XXXIII can be used with benefit. Any system of exercise that actively uses the muscles without the slightest strain can be recommended.

# CHAPTER XII

## PLAIN TALK ABOUT NIGHT LOSSES

Spermatorrhea as manifested in Night Losses — Usually the Result of Youthful Excesses — Not as Serious as Often Supposed.

The belief that involuntary emissions of the seminal fluid during sleep, or " night losses " as they are popularly called, are always productive of grave ailments; that they are a sign of approaching senility, or that they presage insanity and other serious conditions, is, in the main, due to those venders of quack medicine who live by fostering the fears and preying on the ignorance of their dupes, chiefly young men.

As a matter of fact, this impression is far from the truth, for losses of this kind sometimes occur with men who seem to possess superior health and vigor, and, occuring at rare intervals, are not at all as harmful as many suppose. While, of course, an abnormal manifestation of this kind would never occur in one whose health was perfect and whose habits of life were altogether natural; yet in this age of nervous excitement and stimulating food and drink, it would be difficult to find many well sexed men who had not, at some time of life, had losses of semen in this way. They may follow somewhat as the result of a rather full diet, and under such conditions the emission should not occasion any alarm. If not occuring except at extended intervals, very little, if any, debilitating or deleterious consequences should result.

Some physicians even seem to consider them as perfectly natural. We quote the opinion of one:

"Great alarm is often expressed by patients who suffer in this way; but I am enabled to give them much relief when I mention that such emissions, occurring once in every ten or fourteen days, are in the nature of a safety valve, and are even conducive of health in persons who do not take enough exercise and live generously. It would, however, be better for the adult to be free even from these; and I feel convinced that in one who has not allowed himself to dwell on sexual thoughts, but takes strong bodily exercise, and lives abstemiously, emissions will either not occur, or their occurrence may be looked for only very rarely. It is only when the losses or escapes take place repeatedly, attended by symptoms of prostration, with other ill consequences, that the patient should seek medical advice."—*Dr. Acton.*

Of course where the losses are of too frequent occurrence they unquestionably lower the vital powers as a whole, and means should be adopted to lessen their recurrence. Of such means we shall speak later in this chapter.

The excessive nocturnal losses usually

follow on the habit of masturbation. When the victim discovers the terrible consequences to mind and body that attend on self abuse, and regains sufficient strength of will to renounce it, the semen that has been used to supply the artificial demand created by the vice continues to accumulate, and the amorous desires that this creates so influence the brain during sleep that lascivious dreams are produced, which usually result in a loss. Where these dreams are followed by lassitude, dizziness and general weakness, they are occurring too frequently, though it is well to remember the power of mind over body, and that your belief in the debilitating effects of these losses may be influencing your feelings in this way quite seriously. In other words, if you will disabuse your mind of the belief in the extremely injurious effects of these dreams, you may not notice any of the effects which seem so evident when you are anticipating them.

" But when young men are made to believe that any and all emissions are certain and unmistakable indications of coming imbecility, the statement is both preposterous and absurd. Such a statement is wholly unreliable and misleading. After years of acquaintance with men in all periods of life, and after having spoken freely with many upon the subject, the writer is frank to confess that he has yet to meet the first male of the human race, who has passed the period of puberty and who has attained to early manhood, who has not at some time had such emissions, and from whom an undue accumulation of sexual fluid has not passed during hours of sleep in a dream of a more or less amorous nature.

The writer states further:

" We have also carefully examined medical authorities upon this subject, and find that all reliable writers are agreed that such loss of semen, if not occurring at too frequent intervals, is not only quite general, but seemingly natural.''—*Sylvanus Stall, D.D.*

The writer, however, believes that if we all lived perfectly natural and mentally-clean lives, free from all artificial stimulating influences, these emissions would not occur even at extended intervals. If you feel convinced that the losses are becoming excessive, adopt the special rules that follow, at the same time be carefully studying and putting into practice the other general directions for regaining lost strength and vigor that will be found in this work. Do this and you may depend upon securing a complete recovery, although you must remember that it will take time to bring it about. Just how often emissions must occur in order to be considered dangerous is exceedingly difficult to determine. The sexual power of man varies greatly in individuals, and what would be considered excess in one case might be extreme temperance in another. The best plan is to be sure that the symptons of weakness which may follow this loss are not of the imagination, but are a physical reality. When sure of this you can nearly always conclude that the loss is abnormally excessive.

Here then are the specific rules alluded to:

Never sleep on your back. If you are in the habit of doing this, wear a belt with some small article attached to it in such a way that it rests against your spine so that the moment you turn over on your back during sleep you will be awakened by the discomfort occasioned by the arrangement.

Do not under any circumstances neglect to gradually inure yourself to the use of cold water morning and evening, though a complete sitz bath will be found of especial advantage after exercise on rising.

Take up a regular course of exercise, though be very moderate at first. The system illustrated in Chapter XXXII can be recommended.

If the exercise is excessive it will tend to aggravate your trouble. Deep breathing and long walks can be especially commended. A daily walk until thoroughly fatigued will usually aid recovery.

Don't over-eat.

It is a hundred times better to eat too little than to eat too much. Eat nourishing, appetizing foods only—masticate slowly and thoroughly.

Keep the bowels in regular action by using laxative foods, including fruits. If this does not suffice, read chapter on Constipation and follow suggestions given there.

Don't worry.

Don't crowd your brain with lewd thoughts. The more you allow your thoughts to dwell on sexual subjects, the more semen will be accumulated, the more your trouble will be aggravated and the more difficult will be your recovery. Keep the mind pure by directing it on pure things and busy by some active and interesting occupation.

"When the mind is permitted to dwell unduly upon sexual subjects, the secretions become more rapid than is designed, the system is drained, and more injury is done by the impure thought that produces this result than by the dream which attends the emptying of the sacs which are flooded with this vital fluid more rapidly than it can be re-absorbed for use throughout the entire system. Thus it will be seen that the purity of the mind is both of primary and vital importance."—*Sylvanus Stall, D.D.*

Reflect on the nobility and advantages of true manhood and determine to achieve it.

We cannot close this chapter without emphasizing in the strongest possible manner, the fact that the cure of night losses depends largely upon a complete mental reform. Your thoughts must be diverted from everything of a carnal nature. As nearly as you can, you should try to obliterate all thoughts of sex. Do not read books of a nature that are apt to arouse sensual emotions. The moment you find yourself being stirred by reveries of a passionate kind, distract your attention from them by turning to clean and wholesome thoughts.

The daily régime advised in Chapter IX for conquering the habit of self-abuse can be followed with advantage in remedying the trouble under discussion. And remember that although night losses might be termed normal for those who are following the ordinary habits of civilization, which include three hearty meals a day and the use of various condiments and spices which incite one to over-eating, but for a man who keeps himself in perfect health, who exercises frequently, who eats only sufficient food to properly nourish his body, who avoids stimulants of every kind in his dietary, they are certainly abnormal.

## CHAPTER XIII

## DEBILITATING MARITAL EXCESSES

They are the Cause of the Majority of Unhappy Marriages and Keep the Divorce Courts Busy.

One of the most disturbing features of our times is the prevalence of marital troubles. The newspapers are filled with reports of matrimonial miseries and the courts are crowded with suits for separation or divorce. The congenial marriage is the exception, the misfit union the rule. As the home is theoretically the cornerstone of the nation, the matter is one of paramount interest and importance. It appeals to all of us, for, although all are not married, there are few who do not look forward to that condition — or backward at it.

The various theories that are advanced

as to the cause of this same unhappiness by philosophers, social theorists, the clergy, the judiciary, and the cynics throughout the world would fill thousands of volumes. But the writer has often wondered how many of the screeds on the subject expressed the real opinions of the writers. He cannot believe that they fail to see the basic reason of this lamentable state of affairs, or that it is their desire to deceive their readers. But to his mind it is plain that divorces, and the larger majority of the unhappy marriages, are the outcome of abnormal physical conditions induced by sexual excesses, that are largely the result of gross ignorance of those laws with which every adult human being should be familiar, especially those who are in or are about to enter the matrimonial relation.

The majority of married men, and for that matter, women, appear to think and certainly to act as though their sexual powers were limitless. Week after week, month after month, and year after year, they indulge their passions to the extreme limit. The results are always serious. The body is like a chain which is as strong as its weakest link, and when excess of this character becomes continuous the strain on the sexual power link either breaks it or results in the general vigor being gradually undermined. The muscles lose their elasticity, firmness and symmetry; the various vital organs — stomach, heart, lungs — become functionally weaker, and if there is any inherent physical defect or a tendency towards any disease, the condition of the body is favorable to its development. Thousands of persons have died and are still dying of consumption and other wasting diseases which are made possible because of the lowering of the vitality and the consequent lessening of the power of resistance to disease brought about by excesses committed in the name of matrimony.

" In Nature, sexual intercourse has but one aim, and that is procreation. This act, which is one of the greatest mysteries of life, and should be reverenced as a sacrament, should be performed only for the purpose of securing offspring. Every other such act, or sexual excitement, constitutes vice, undermines health, and is a sacrilege against nature's laws ordained by God Almighty. For the purpose of procreation, one act may suffice; then, while the fruit is developing, and also during the time of nursing, the mother should abstain. This state of affairs we find with all wild animals."—*A. F. Reinhold, Ph.D., M.D.*

The entire conventional idea of marriage and the duties of a wife to her husband is based on perverted theories that have done much towards bringing about the unsatisfactory matrimonial conditions that are now almost universal. The marriage ceremony is supposed to give a man every privilege he may desire. In other words, that it permits him to gratify his lust without let or hindrance. The wife is presumed to be subjected to his every wish. The laws of nature, or the laws of God, warrant no such conclusion. The truth is that the wishes of the wife should be paramount—that the husband should be subject to and controlled by her in sexual matters. When this outrage on married women that is the outcome of the assumption of their total subjection to men in marital life, is fully realized, one of the principal causes of diseases peculiar to the sex and its matrimonial unhappiness in general will be understood and probably modified if not removed altogether.

While man is much to blame for the unsatisfactory conditions that follow most marriages, woman is not altogether faultless in the matter, for it is her privilege and duty to regulate sexual affairs. She should possess a strongly defined feminine instinct which should clearly indicate her course of action. If she does not possess this instinct, she has not the slightest right to marry. And if possessed of it, and the husband refuses to be guided thereby the couple may just as well separate immediately, for no happiness will ever be found in a marriage under such conditions.

If separation does not take place, the so-called marriage is like an engine without a governor, a ship without a rudder. Excess that is limited only by the exhaustion of the physical forces of the pair can rarely be avoided. And with such excess comes all sorts of ills and weaknesses peculiar to woman. The man, too, feels exhausted, worn-out and debilitated. His energies, so continually needed to carry on his business, or to assist him in reaching the goal of his ambitions, are wasted in excesses that only end when the vital powers are dissipated or the repulsion comes on that is born of satiety.

How many thousands of young women, apparently in good health, enter the realms of matrimony, and as a result of a short sojourn therein find that their health of body and mind is being sacrificed. The cause is always the same — an undeveloped sexual instinct, and the perverted impression, either on the part of one or both, that marriage means total subjection to the wishes of another. On the rocks of this false conclusion are shattered the happiness, health and future prospects of thousands of married couples. Herein, too, lies the paramount importance of superb physical health. Notwithstanding the influence that may be brought to bear on a woman by others or by what she may be assured is her duty, she will not stoop to anything that will outrage her instincts if she possesses all the power, beauty and health that are among the constituents of true womanhood.

Such a woman is perfectly balanced and

will not violate such balance by yielding to the undue desires of a husband whose actions are due to lust and not to love.

"Woman is the final umpire as to its frequency. Following her lead will usually conduct all to matrimonial harmony; ignoring it, to discord. *Only a healthy one, however, will decide right.* A husband who tenderly loves a delicate wife will find no difficulty in being continent, because he loves her too well to subject her to what would be injurious. Attempts have been made by legislators and divines to fix definitely a limit to the conjugal approaches which should be binding upon all, but this is evidently impracticable. Generally speaking the hygienic rule is, that after the act the person should feel well and strong, the sleep should be sound, and the mind clear. Whenever this is not the case, when the limbs feel languid, the appetite feeble or capricious, the head ache, the intellect dull, and the faculties sluggish, then there certainly is excess, and the act should be indulged in more rarely. Those who strictly observe these rules will need no others, and will incur no danger from over-indulgence."—*Prof. O. S. Fowler.*

It is not hard to understand why marital intemperance so saps the physical and nervous powers, making its devotee a peevish, ambitionless, unhappy creature, a failure in the commercial life, a pessimist abroad and a nuisance at home. It is because he is a spendthrift of his most valuable bodily treasure,—the seminal fluid. Itself the source of life, it is distilled from his life, and its reckless squandering means that he is throwing away his life.

Some physiologists claim that one drop of semen is equal to sixty drops of blood. Although it would be difficult to determine accurately the relative physiological values of the vital fluid and the blood, no one will question the richness of the former in vital elements. It contains the very essence of a man, for is it not bone of his bone, flesh of his flesh?

The reader will probably and very properly ask for a definition of excess. How often can one indulge in sexual intercourse and still keep within the bounds of temperance? No hard and fast restrictions can be imposed on a body of married people. No one rule can be made for everybody. Each man must find out for himself just what his capabilities are, for what would be termed excessive in one case might be considered temperate in another.

Nevertheless, even when the parties to a marriage are of vigorous health, when both are well sexed and both are of an amorous disposition, excesses will and must tell in the long run. Nature will not be imposed upon. If you defy nature's legislation, you are a law-breaker in her eyes and no bloodhound that ever put nose to trail is more implacable in pursuit of a wrongdoer than is nature unless you come back to her by the ways by which you left her, retracing your steps thereon.

"Many married people will give themselves up to the embrace daily, often more than once, and that for years. But not only its frequency, but the manner in which it is performed, are so unnatural and studiously licentious that the most desperate cases of paralysis and epilepsy are frequently the direct and immediate result. Locomotor ataxia and palsy, too, often follow in its wake."—*A. T. Reinhold, Ph.D., M.D.*

The most reliable guides are your own feelings if you are really anxious to know if you are giving way to excesses. When living in the marital relation and you seem to be lacking in energy, when your strength appears to be steadily lessening, when that "tired feeling" becomes chronic, and if you are coincidently taking regular exercise, a nourishing, wholesome diet, proper bathing, and insuring yourself a copious supply of pure air, you can at once conclude that sexual excess has much, if not all, to do with your weakness.

Of course, the remedy under these circumstances is temperance, or preferably entire abstinence from sexual relations. In addition to this abstinence every possible natural means for building up the physical forces, as advised later in this book, must be used regularly and perseveringly.

Men and women, according to the poet, are " but children of a larger growth." Be that as it may, it is certain that at every stage of their lives they need special schooling of some sort or the other, and never more so than when they are on the verge of matrimony to teach them to avoid those things that are responsible for the query, " Is marriage a failure? "

Sexual temperance is about all that can be expected from the average married couple, but if the rules of life that carry with them the highest degree of mental and physical power are followed, sexual privileges will be accorded to the husband only at periods when procreation is prepared for and expected. This exalted code of morals, the following of which leads to the highest human happiness, is described very fully in the writer's book entitled, Marriage a Life-Long Honeymoon.

# CHAPTER XIV

## ALCOHOL KILLS VIRILITY

### The Use of this Stimulant Excites Lust and Destroys Manhood.

Next to the excesses already recited, the greatest harm accrues to sexual virility through the use of alcohol. The powers for evil possessed by this poison are of a dual nature for it is not only an inciter to excesses and so is responsible for the ills which are the outcome of them, but it is also a direct cause in itself of loss of manhood.

The preservation of the species being, as it would seem, the first duty or law of nature, it has been so ordered that every faculty or function shall be enlisted in its observance. It is for this reason that the sexual instinct is of so overmastering a kind that it possesses every part and particle of a man, mentally and physically.

Now it follows that if one or several of the powers that should assist in the act of intercourse is below par in any way, consummation, wholly or to an extent, is prevented and in any event the beauty, significance and enjoyment of the act is not made known to the imperfect participant. For this reason he who indulges in alcoholic drinks may have his desires inordinately increased thereby, but he can never satisfy them, because that which has created them has murdered the means of assuaging them.

" It is scarcely necessary that we should say anything about the injurious effects of liquors of all kinds upon the reproductive organs. It is well known that drunkards and tipplers are easily robbed of sexual power. The ancient proverb says, ' Venus is drowned in Bacchus.' Shakespeare aptly displays his marvelous range of information in the play 'Macbeth,' where the porter says to Macduff, 'Drinking provokes the desire, but it takes away the performance; it makes him, and it mars him; it sets him on, and it takes him off; it persuades him, and it disheartens him,' etc. Manliness and virile power in their best development are impossible to those who use liquor of any kind in any quantity."—*Sylvanus Stall, D.D.*

Another writer puts the subject even more emphatically:

"The generative organs in a sense suffer more in proportion from the undue use of alcohol, than any other organs of the body. This is because their normal, healthy action calls for the combined assistance of all the other forces and parts of the body. In the instance of the hard drinker, the harm done to his nervous system and to his muscular economy culminates in the organs alluded to, in the shape of the whole or partial paralysis of their powers."

And again:

"The inveterate rum-drinker is, in the course of time so affected by his vice that he is reduced to the physical level of an eunuch in the harem of an Eastern potentate. The man who is given over to the alcohol habit is being as certainly deprived of his manhood as if he were undergoing an operation by the surgeon's knife for that purpose."

The sexual organs in order to be in a healthy condition must be kept plentifully and steadily supplied with good blood. The effect of alcohol upon the circulation is well known. It deadens or numbs the many nerves of the heart including the inhibitory or restraining nerves, the result being that for some time there is an excessive flow of blood to the organs, followed by a reaction and simultaneously the system is called upon to supply the extra energy needed under the influence of a poisonous stimulant. So we have an interference with the nervous system, an irregular supply of poisoned blood, a draft on the reserve vitality and a harming of the digestive apparatus, all affecting our sexual powers at one and the same time.

"Alcohol and other narcotics deaden the nerves and so diminish their action. This effect first shows itself in the nerves which control the passage of the blood through the small arteries. If the use of alcohol is continued until the habit of drinking is formed, the derangement of the nerves becomes more marked. The nerves lose control of the muscles, and all the organs of the body become more or less out of order because the nerves that ought to produce harmony of action are practically paralyzed."

Yet another authority remarks:

"Along with sexual health and calmness go good general health and general quietness of the nerves. Nothing is so detrimental to this condition as the use of stimulants and narcotics."—Prof. O. S. Fowler.

No true strength can be produced by any stimulant. It is always false strength, is created at the expense of vital power, and assists just that much in lessening the real strength of all parts of the body as it gives momentary fictitious strength.

"If a drinking man should measure the strength of his muscles, that is, the weight he can lift before and after an alcoholic drink is taken, he would find he could lift less after the dram than before. He may think he can lift more, but the test will prove that he cannot. The tipsy man often boasts of his strength until his limbs are scarcely able to sustain him, because the alcohol he has taken has so deadened his nerves of feeling that he does not know his real condition."—*Lessons in Hygiene.*

And it may be added that the drunkard has an exaggerated idea of his sexual strength, usually to his harm and always to his disappointment.

It cannot be too often repeated that physical vigor and sexual vigor are companions. You will always find them together in the same person. Anything that tends to build up one will increase the power of the other. Therefore take a lesson from prize-fighters and other athletes who when training for a contest, which means training to the end of attaining the highest degree of health, leave all stimulants absolutely alone.

The practice of taking a " nip " before meals is most harmful. The " nip " first creates a false appetite, then kills it, leaving in its place a craving for more stimulants instead of a desire for good, wholesome food. The result is ruination to the digestive organs and a contingent lowering of the sexual powers, for it stands to reason that a poorly nourished body cannot properly nourish any of its organs or functions.

" There are some substances upon which the gastric juices have no action or, if any, certainly not the power of converting them into nutriment, and alcohol is one of them. Digestion being one of the most important of all of the bodily economy, it is indispensable to the due performance of all the other functions. Consequently when it becomes impaired the whole system languishes and all of the functions become affected also." —*Dr. Thomas Sewell.*

One of the most terrible of the many counts against the sot is, however, that he or she is very likely to bequeath the love of alcohol to offspring. Like the poison of syphilis, the poison of alcohol can be inherited by posterity and with almost equally appalling results. Heavy indeed is the responsibility of the parent who leaves such a cursed legacy to a child.

" We say a child looks like his father.

That resemblance may not be confined to the face alone; brain, nerves and other organs may be as much like the father's as is the face. Alcohol will shrivel the nerves and brain of the drinking parent, weaken his will, sear and blunt his conscience, and give him a craving appetite for more alcohol. It will make him coarse, cruel and brutal. As the face of the child may look like the face of the parent, so the child may inherit all or any of the conditions that alcohol produced in the parent."—*Eugene Bouton, Ph.D.*

" It is not merely the man or woman inflamed by alcohol — at or near the time of sexual intercourse — that implants the fatal disease in the child at the very moment of conception; not this and these only; but they are equally guilty, perhaps more so, who,— with their blood diseased from long saturation with this poison, their nervous system shattered, and the very foundations of their being tainted,— pro-

ceed deliberately to engender offspring."
— *Albert Day, M.D.*

Of the power of alcohol to incite to lust allusion has already been made. It is said that over two thousand cases of rape recorded in this country last year were attempted or consummated by men under the influence of liquor. It is the favorite instrument of the libertine who seeks to rob the virtuous of her virtue. The groggery is never far removed from the brothel. And marital excesses of all sorts are but too often the outcome of the wine-laden dinner, or the " small bottle " of the theatre supper.

" Persons whose arteries are filled with blood, poisoned and corrupted by alcohol, will be possessed with a mania for lust. Husbands who drink the poison draught are apt to prove faithless to their marriage vows. Wives who drink to intoxication want only opportunity to commit adultery. No married person can long put faith in a drunken companion."—*Charles A. Story, M.D., in Alcohol, Its Nature and Effects.*

"If this process (the drinking of alcoholic beverages) is often repeated, the lower propensities are strengthened by use until by and by they act of their own accord, while the moral restraining powers or will, weakened by disuse or induced diseases, are practically nullified. The man is no longer under the control of his voluntary power, but is under the dominion of his lower appetites, and they are as much beyond his control as is the beating of his heart. In short, alcohol excites the animal nature to powerful and ungovernable activity and utterly paralyzes reason, conscience and will."—*Nathan Allen, M.D.*

The method of treatment for ridding one's self of the enslaving habit is within the power of every man who has the least amount of will power left within him. Read carefully the chapter on Diet; follow conscientiously the instructions as to exercise, bathing, clothing, fresh air, etc., etc.

After you have begun to observe these rules lessen by one every day or every other day the number of drinks you are in the habit of taking. When you are at length taking only one each day, try to make it one every other day, then one every third day, after which you will probably find no difficulty in leaving alcohol alone altogether. The better way, however, is to break off the habit at once. The desire for a stimulant of any kind always indicates a lowered condition of the system in general. But when the natural means indicated for building up the physical forces begin to assert themselves but little difficulty will be found in doing this. The importance of never overeating, and not to eat at any time unless very hungry, cannot be too strongly emphasized.

One of the main causes of the craving for a stimulant is over-eating, and this fact must be clearly understood if you are desirous of ridding yourself of the slavery of drink. You cannot hope to own the delicacy and joy of this superb power unless the benumbing influence of alcohol is totally withdrawn.

"The use of liquor destroys health, disfigures the body, ruins the nervous system, dethrones the reason, produces insanity, becomes the parent of idiocy; it blunts the finer feelings and sensibilities; it fills our poor-houses with paupers and crowds our prisons with criminals; it breaks the hearts of parents and pauperizes helpless women and innocent children; it leads to vice and violence, and plunges its victims into temporal and eternal ruin."—*Sylvanus Stall, D.D.*

# CHAPTER XV

## TOBACCO A FOE TO MANLY VIGOR

### It Dopes the Nervous System and Ruins the Digestion.

Nicotine, an oily liquid, the active principle of tobacco, is an alkaloid poison. When administered in sufficient quantities it causes death. In smaller doses it has a direct and numbing effect on the brain and nerves. Its use causes an undue flow of saliva which is in itself a strain on the system and the beginning of stomach troubles. It is also a gastric irritant. It may be absorbed by being taken into the lungs by the inhalation of tobacco smoke or through contact with the mucous membrane of the mouth with the aid of a cigar or pipe.

There is a uniformity of opinion among writers on the subject as to the effects of tobacco on sexual powers. The author has heard of numerous cases where tobacco has been the direct cause of impotence. One case in particular is remembered where a patient was being treated for an entire loss of power induced by the "weed." The physician had prescribed the usual remedies, and had been attending the patient for some time without any sign of improvement being made manifest. One day while reading a work on the evil results of smoking, he was surprised to note the special injury which the author of the work claimed that smoking produced on the sexual powers. While he already realized that the results of smoking were far from desirable, he did not consider them as injurious as they were claimed to be. Then it was, however, that he remembered that the patient whom he was treating was a great smoker, and that he had told him on one or two occasions that his improvement might be more rapid if he would be moderate in the habit.

That which he had read appealed to him strongly, however, and he determined to enjoin entire abstinence from smoking upon his patient and to watch the result. In less than a month the sick man's long-lost powers returned. The physician then allowed him to resume his cigars. The result was that in a short time the old trouble re-appeared, and ultimately he found that cigars must be avoided or else a chronic condition of impotence would ensue.

The use of tobacco, either by smoking or chewing, has an enormous influence on the nervous system. Nothing proves this so emphatically as the intense, almost overpowering, craving for a smoke or chew which is one of the many lamentable consequences that attend the use of the weed after it has become a habit. It benumbs and destroys the finer sensibility of the nerves. Any influence on the general nervous system of course affects the organs of sex directly, for, as explained before, they are a most delicate part of the nervous system itself.

"The depressing effect of nicotine on the nerve centres is most marked. An excessive user of tobacco is almost always a person of bilious or saturnine temperament. And it will usually be found that his vitality is of a much lower order than that of a person who is a non-smoker. Nicotine is terribly destructive of nervous force."—*Silas M. Briely, M.D.*

"The general use of tobacco diminishes nervous action. It is a substance which enters into the system without furnishing it with any needed element. It has a particularly paralyzing effect upon the nerves which control the muscles of the heart and other important organs."

Smoking, or the use of tobacco in any form, therefore, must be avoided if a combination of strength and nerve force is desired. The resultant vigor carries with it all the intensity and power of superb sexual power as has already been stated in this work.

" To one who has not attained his entire growth, the use of tobacco stunts the body and dwarfs the muscles, making them flabby and weak. When used to excess, tobacco greatly affects the vision. Physicians who make the treatment of the eye a specialty tell us that when they use the magnifying lens, and throw the light in upon the retina of the eye, they can tell immediately when one is addicted to the excessive use of tobacco. It also deadens the hearing, greatly affects the heart, producing palpitation, and when used regularly, in large quantities, results in producing what is called " tobacco heart." The results of either smoking or chewing can often be noticed in its effects upon the nerves, rendering the individual both nervous and irritable, even under small provocation. Surgeons tell us that their experience in the operating room has developed the fact that men who are addicted to the use of tobacco quite generally suffer a lack of manly fortitude, and are noticeably cowardly under the severe trial of a surgical operation. Tobacco discolors the teeth, makes the breath offensive, excites the glands which secrete the saliva, and tends to produce dyspepsia, low spirits, a pale face, and an emanciated form. It also tends to produce dizziness, rush of blood to the head, palpitation of the heart, loss of memory, and a diseased condition of the mouth. Such results have been noted in the death of prominent persons, such as General Grant, and many others."—*Sylvanus Stall, D.D.*

One of the most convincing arguments against the use of tobacco is the fact that all athletes in training entirely avoid it. No matter how much they have been addicted to the habit, when the time arrives for them to begin the work which is to key their bodies up to the highest pitch of manly health and strength, smoking is immediately and absolutely tabooed. The effect of tobacco on physical endurance is most marked, as a smoker, just like a hard drinker, will after one or two strenuous efforts be entirely exhausted by efforts that do not try the non-smoker at all.

Nicotine, like alcohol and sexual excess, is productive of strange results in the human system. The writer has known of apparent cases of rheumatism, glandular diseases, chronic neuralgia, cancerous affections, and even mental failure being brought about by tobacco. All disappeared when the smoker quit his pet vice.

"A poisonous substance like tobacco, cannot be brought frequently into contact with an absorbing surface like the mucous membrane, without in many cases producing disorders of the system which the smoker is probably quite ready to attribute to any other cause than that which would render it necessary for him to deprive himself of what he erroneously considers to be an article necessary to his existence."—*Dr. B. J. Taylor.*

The most harmful and nauseating form in which tobacco is used is the cigarette. In the case of the cigar or pipe, the smoke is almost always taken into the mouth, kept there for a brief space and then blown away. But the cigarette fiend invariably inhales. That is, he deliberately draws the pugent, sickening fumes into his lungs. Naturally the cells of those organs which bring the blood into contact with the inhaled air, take up a portion of the smoke, including more or less of the vapor of nicotine and burnt paper. The blood is instantly poisoned, the nerve centres acutely affected, and the general tone of the system lowered. Also, as is always the case where cigarettes are used, the mental and moral natures of the man are frightfully distorted and so the cigarette to a very great extent breeds our supply of criminals, including sexual perverts.

"The statistics of crime in the Metropolis prove conclusively that the great majority of criminals are addicted to the use of cigarettes. There seems to be some indissoluble bond between the thief, the thug, and the swindler and the 'coffin nail.'"—*Dr. A. J. Priestly in Prison Records.*

Allusion has already been made in the power for evil exercised by tobacco on sexual virility. Unfortunately, not only does the slave of the weed suffer himself, but he entails much of his weakness on his offspring. Here again nicotine and alcohol have much in common. Any family physician will tell you that the children of a confirmed smoker are rarely all that they ought to be. They are living and pathetic protests against the misuse of the weed. In the case of the cigarette victim, however, the evil is magnified tenfold.

"I observed that the children of these (Cuban cigarmakers) were very scrawny and feeble. A brother physician resident in Havana, said that both mothers and fathers smoked cigarettes incessantly and that many babies were born with all the symptoms of incipient nicotine poisoning. Also that the percentage of still born infants and miscarriages were enormous. He attributed all these unhappy conditions to the excessive use of tobacco."—*J. W. Hobley, M.D., in Notes on Cuba.*

A well-known New York physician who, through his connection with one of the institutions in question was for some years closely identified with the people of the Ghetto, was asked why the invariably healthy Hebrew lad usually became a puny, spiritless, sallow-skinned man. He answered:

"Outside of the sweat-shop, the cigarette is the curse of the East Side. Go down Grand Street, during lunch hour, and the youth or man who hasn't one of the coffin nails between his lips is a curiosity there. These fellows smoke from breakfast time to bedtime, and in scores of cases I've known them to get up in the middle of the night to satisfy their craving. The average cigarette is bad enough, but those sold in New York's Jewish quarter are made of the vilest tobacco, or of chopped 'snipes'—cigar butts—picked up in the gutters. The cigarettes can be bought three or four for a cent, so you can imagine just what they are. I attribute at least thirty-three per cent. of East Side crime to its detestable cigarettes. From the moment a man becomes a cigarette fiend he ceases to be normal, and then anything is possible to him in the way of criminality. The diseases—especially those of a mental type—bred by the East Side cigarette are numberless. I believe that it is only the sturdy constitutions of the women that prevents the cigarette from causing the Ghetto to become a colony of idiots or weaklings."

For the average smoker, however, it is a comparatively easy matter to break the bonds of tobacco if the same methods are adopted as advised for curing the liquor habit — that is among other things, to gradually lessen the use of it day by day. Remember too, to faithfully follow the instructions for re-constructing the nervous and muscular powers for they are of just as much help in ridding one of the smoking or chewing habit as they are in the cure of the alcohol habit. If you desire to be young again, if you long to experience the joy, elasticity and exuberance that accompany extreme virility, value that virility when regained and foreswear the use of tobacco while life endures.

## CHAPTER XVI

# SIN OF SEXUAL STARVATION

### Those Who Practice it are mostly Egotists or Fanatics.

Human egotism takes strange shapes. One form of it consists of a disposition to criticize the methods of the Almighty in regard to sexuality. The persons afflicted with this type of dementia — for that's what it amounts to — look with disfavor on those provisions of Nature which have for their end the establishing of home centres and the procreation of the race. They seem to think that sex is improper and marriage more or less shocking. Of such a sort was the woman who remarked that she thought it rather indelicate of God to allow babies to be born without clothing. Another of the kind is said to have asserted that she detested the French language because it contained no neuter gender which to her mind was the gender par excellence.

These persons whom Macaulay aptly nicknamed " prurient prudes " go through life with their noses uplifted sniffing foul air where others only smell sweet odors. If they see a piece of exquisitely carved, nude statuary they ignore the art and beauty of it and declaim against its unclad condition. The frank innocence of childhood is to them only an evidence of original sin. They detect double meanings where the normal individual can see but a sincere sentiment. Love is merely a veiled form of lust so they aver and the sacredness and nobility of marriage are lost upon them.

As stated, the false attitude of these unhappy creatures is usually the outcome of a diseased egotism. They succeed in persuading themselves and try to persuade others that they are possessed of superlative refinement that prompts them to shudder at such gross things as matrimony and parentage. Those wonderful organs upon which Nature has expended so much care and attention, together with the group of powers and emotions that are identified with them, are all a portion of our lower nature according to the superior persons in question. And the " lower nature " is something to blush to think about, to be crushed, ignored, put out of sight and kept out of sight like any other improper thing. In short, so these narrow gauge prudes declare, the things of sex are as vulgar as they are embarrassing and as unnecessary as both.

Of course there are individuals who, while fairly normal, conscientiously believe that a state of continence is the ideal state if not for mankind at large, at least as far as they are concerned. Sometimes such persons have the power of living out their beliefs like Pere Hyacinthe and Honoré de Balzac. At other times the theory observes for a season and then Nature asserts herself as Gibbon, in The Decline and Fall of the Roman Empire, tells us that it did in the case of the early Christians who put their virtue to too extreme tests. But continence based upon alleged conscience is comparatively rare. The truth is that the man of healthful conscience marries because he knows that if he fails to do so he is sinning greatly against nature and himself.

Like " cranks " in general, the crank that proposes a life-long sexual fast is not content to starve himself but desires the world to starve also. Here again we see the ear marks of the egotist whose dearest wish it always is that people should pander to his vanity by attempting to follow his example.

Even if the anti-sex people were but partially right which they are not, it would be impossible to lay down hard and fast rules. Because of our abnormal condition no two are exactly alike. That which means happiness to one may mean abject misery to another. In every species of animal outside of the human animal there exists a certain degree of uniformity in physique and mentality; but the physical and mental traits and powers of men are as widely different as are the quickness, suppleness and mental acuteness of the tiger, far removed from the clumsiness, apparent stupidity, and phlegmatic temperament of the hippopotamus. With this fact clear, would any intelligent person dare to lay down rules for all to follow indiscriminately, especially on the vital questions of sex?

When the body demands food and cannot get it, the resulting starvation makes itself evident on form and feature in an unmistakable manner. So too when there is a love famine, when the attempt is made to crush sex, the unsatisfied needs of the mind and physical being are shown in every act and expression of the person undergoing the experience.

Contrast the appearance of a spinster who has spent much of her life in declaiming against the "lower nature" of her fellows with that of a young matron who has a brood of youngsters around her. In the first case, there is usually a spare, angular figure, a parchment-like, lantern-jawed countenance, a scrawny neck, and an acidity of tongue and expression. The chief occupation of the prude — scandal — is hers. She looks the vinegary superfluity that she is and the world is none the better for her living and none the poorer for her passing away.

In the second instance, the wife and mother, if her marriage is reasonably happy, is cheery, healthy, plump usually, winsome invariably, surrounded by an atmosphere of restful domesticity, charitable to all, happy in the love of her husband and children and blessed with a sense of duties fulfilled and a life well lived. And all this the outcome of a well nourished, not starved, sexual nature.

Sins of omission are not less harmful in their results than are sins of commission. Especially is this so when the non-use of the love nature is involved. Not only, as in the case of the spinster just cited, is the evil of a personal nature, but the Maker intended that the sexual powers should be used to the end of invoking from out the unknown spaces the souls and bodies of little children. When the sin of omission has been enacted in regard to these it is questionable if the refusal to bring into existence a life is not morally, just as much murder as is the taking of a life. It need hardly be added that this assertion applies to the prudes and duty-shirkers of both sexes.

There is another aspect to the matter also. The sexual impulse, if prevented from acting in a normal fashion, is apt to make itself manifest in grotesque or unnatural shapes. Of these last we will not speak at length. Suffice it to say that physicians who make a specialty of the treatment of mental disorders, of nervous diseases, or of sexual "eccentricities," can tell strange and terrible stories of some of those who, possessed of original normal sexuality, tried to ignore its meaning and its use. The sin of attempted sexual annihilation hatched other sins of which it were not well to allude. Of the grotesque form of the same thing one illustration is all that is needed. Can anything be more sickeningly humorous than the sight of an elderly virgin cuddling and cooing over and caressing a wheezy pug dog whose nose, upon which she is imprinting fervent kisses, has in all likelihood been investigating the neighboring lamp posts for a block or so!

Another manner in which Nature shows

her displeasure at these sterile lives is by taking from them the magnetism and charm that nearly always accompany a person of a high degree of health and vitality. These disappear, and there remains a vacancy in their places. The consequent dullness of looks and demeanor of the victims is most noticeable and proclaims their lack of sexual and general physical stamina, while it additionally indicates that they are neither men nor women, but mere nonentities, from a sexual standpoint.

In the proportion that one succeeds in crushing out what is thus erroneously and absurdly called the "lower nature," to a similar degree will one's powers deteriorate in other ways. A man, for instance, to be of any importance must first *be a man,* and without that stamina, energy and wholesome vigor which is the accompaniment of finely sexed manhood, there is but small prospect of his ever accomplishing anything of importance in life. Instead of adopting those means that theoretically or possibly lessen the powers of sex, it is the plain duty of every man to try to build and retain strength of that character. Its possession makes him more manly, more courageous, and more capable of rising above the level of mediocrity.

There is not the slightest occasion to fear that one can acquire sexual strength which will grow beyond control. There is always greater power of control under normal than there is under abnormal conditions. Normal vitality is steady, healthy — nothing unnatural or feverish about it. Often under some momentary stimulus even weak organs acquire an unnatural strength, which always react to their disadvantage by bringing about a relapse that not infrequently deprives them of power for a time. But the man of sound body and mind may rest assured that the latter will always work in harmony with the former and that both will never permit of weakness or allow of the indulgence of undue desire.

To sum up, sexual starvation is sin. The legitimate gratification of the sexual appetite at the period when procreation is prepared for and desired is virtue.

Everything in Nature emphasizes the necessity of marriage; animal and vegetable life everywhere gives evidence to that effect. The highest degree of attainable physical perfection can never be acquired unless the mated condition is secured at the proper period of life. It may be put off; the day of its consummation may be delayed; but it should come before the powers of manhood and womanhood are on the wane, or the participants will never be able to taste its joys and reap its benefits to the same extent that they could during the brightness and strength of full maturity.

Successful men nearly always marry; many of them are fathers of large families.

The founding of a home with one for whom there exists an ardent yet reverential love, is usually one of the first steps to fame and fortune. It makes one feel settled in life. It directs one's efforts towards a definite goal. The seriousness and responsibilities of home life give strength to the will and persistence in life's aims while the solitary man or woman drifts towards they know not what like a compassless ship in an uncharted sea.

"Loves and marriages are common to all nature. They exist between atom and atom and we call it attraction; between element and element and the chemist names it affinity; between iron and the magnet, and it is christened magnetism. But it is marriage nevertheless."—*Dr. Mason Good.*

"The early and faithful union of one man with one woman is the true ideal of society. Such secures the health and purity of the family relation and is the foundation of society and national welfare. It is supported by sound principles of physiology, by historical study of the rise and fall of the nations and by a consideration of the evils of our present age."—*Elizabeth Blackwell, M.D.*

# CHAPTER XVII

## SEXUAL PERVERSITY

The Most Revolting of Any Form of Depraved Passion Usually Results from Bestial Excesses.

When any faculty or function of our bodies becomes abnormally developed it is at the expense of its fellow faculties and we are in consequence mentally or physically unbalanced as the case may be. If the faculty so enlarged belongs to the higher part of our natures the result is the poet, the scientist, or the successful evangelist. That "great wit to madness closely is allied" is generally admitted.

If, however, the lower part is affected we have the notorious criminal, the successful libertine or, it may be, that moral monster with which this chapter deals — the sexual pervert. And if this last has a place in the economy of Nature, as even the most loathsome of her creatures has, it is to point the moral in regard to the results and possibilities of sexual excesses. For the pervert is, above all, the offspring of such excesses, a child of the unbridled lust that breeds despair, madness and death.

In the majority of books of this type it is the fashion to ignore the subject with which this chapter deals, through motives of alleged modesty. Yet the surgeon who declined to lance a pus-laden abscess on the plea that it wasn't nice to handle or pleasant to look upon, would certainly receive the ridicule and contempt which he deserved. And so the author feels that he too would be worthy of just condemnation were he to refrain from passing on that hideous ulcer of civilization, the moral degenerate or, to use the plainer term, the sexual pervert.

While there are no excuses for the ordinary sexual sinners, there is at least a sort of explanation of their actions. The man or woman who lends himself or herself to legal prostitution on the loveless marriage bed or to hardly less blamable acts of promiscuous intercourse, is but following a natural if misdirected instinct. The same remark stands good for persons who insist on indulging their carnal appetites at periods when Nature plainly forbids their so doing. And even the wretched victim of self abuse, while polluting body and jeopardizing soul, usually allows the imagination to run riot sexually.

But the hideous mystery of sexual perversion, who shall attempt to make it clear? It violates the fundamental principle of Creation — the attraction of sex to sex. It is the carrion fruit of a putrid mentality. It outrages in filthy fashion the laws of man and God. It is devoid of the questionable attractiveness with which many sins are clothed and instead, is a shape of repulsive horror. Saint Decuman held that it was the "unpardonable sin" of Scripture.

The curse of outraged Nature is upon it for the degenerate almost always fills a suicide's grave or a cell in an insane asylum.

Before touching on its causes and thereby suggesting its prevention if not its cure, let it be said that the pervert of both sexes is as old as history itself, and, as intimated, invariably the product of civilization. The Bible, not being possessed of the monkish prudishness of our modern teachers, uses plain terms in connection with the vice. Sodom and Gomorrah, the cities of the Plain, were destroyed by a rain of fire because of one species of pervert that swarmed within their walls. Death by stoning was the lot of the pervert under Mosaic law. The Persians of old shot him to death with burning arrows. Among the ancient Greeks and just when the canker of luxury was eating into the vitals of the national life, perverts of divers types abounded and a peculiarly disgusting sort of degenerate vice formed a portion of the religious rites in more than one temple in Athens. In Rome in the days of her decline, perverts were accorded a semi-social recognition. The disastrous endings of some of the Crusades were attributed to the unnatural vices and simultaneous moral and physical degeneracy of the wearers of the cross, such vices being learned by them from the Saracens. To-day, the hotbeds of the evil are those Oriental nations which, once powerful and world conquering, are now but the emasculated shadows of their former selves. But present day nations, and, to our shame and sorrow be it said, this country, are infested by the pervert also, and to what an increasing extent only those who have been brought into official or professional touch with him, or for that matter, her, can appreciate. But an instance or two will suffice. Not so long since it was publicly reported that the detectives of a certain precinct came to the conclusion that a certain ferry house was the rendezvous of a horde of these indescribable creatures. Within three days twenty-two arrests, all young men, were made, the evidence in each instance being of an irreputable nature. Two of the prisoners, both members of wealthy families, committed suicide. A detective informed me that recently there existed on Houston street in New York city a resort given over to the accommodation of the votaries of the vice. Slummers knew it well, together with its crowd of unsexed things that spoke in falsetto voices and called each other by girls names. Further uptown were and for that matter still are " clubs " whose members are all degenerates and whose semi-annual balls, at which the hosts and guests are men, three-fourths of whom wear women's dress, are familiar to New York " rounders."

Apart from these — the aristocrats of their nauseous class — are the shoals of painted, perfumed, Kohl-eyed, lisping, mincing youths that at night swarm on Broadway in the Tenderloin section, or haunt the parks and 5th avenue, ogling every man that passes and — it is pleasant to relate — occasionally getting a sound thrashing or an emphatic kicking. Then there are the degenerates in private life, the majority of whom are wealthy and not infrequently members of the learned professions. A large percentage of such are men of middle life or well up in years. Sometimes, through a hint in the newspapers, the public gets a glimpse into the interior of such whited sepulchres, but for the most part only the police, the reporters and the physicians know the appalling number of perverts who are prominent in church affairs, in social circles and who are men of family. Incidentally, it may be added that a certain New York physician, who died a few years ago, left an estate of over a million dollars. He made a specialty of treating wealthy men and women for "sexual abberation," as he chose to call it, and employed three assistants.

Experts are pretty generally agreed in that the perversion of the sexual instinct may be brought about in several ways. Many authorities allege that it can be induced by pre-natal influences. A woman who is pregnant may doom her unborn child to a life of nameless infamy if she permits her passions to overcome her to the extent of indulging in delerious caresses and unchecked lust. Her mate will of course be a partner in the crime, but through the medium of his actions is likely to vary the terrible results.

Again the continuous unbridled relation of one sex with the other sex breeds perverts. Normal or legitimate passion is kept alive by a certain amount of restraint being imposed upon it. Physical considerations, respect for oneself or for one's wife, or husband, or a recognition of the laws of nature all tend to the prevention of excess and the retention of normality. But where none of these exist satiety is bound to follow. The lustful desires remain, but they cannot be satisfied by natural means. The nerves of passion have been so overtaxed that they are in a paralyzed state and refuse to respond unless they are spurred into activity by extraordinary methods. So the victim of his appetites seeks from the abnormal that which the normal can no longer give him — a stimulus to his sensuality. And so we have the perverts that grow from the cloying pleasures of the harems of the East or the harems of Paris, London or New York.

Sexual perverts are also found in bodies of men who are by force of circumstances prevented from enjoying the companionship of women. Armies in the field, crews of ships on long voyages, and so forth, breed many perverts. Among the semi-civilized nations of the East that either lead a life of almost constant warfare or have polyandry as an institution, perverts are very common. The travellers, the late Colonel Burnaby and H. Savage Landor, testify to as much. Boarding schools or other influences or surroundings which tempt the boy or youth to masturbation may tempt him also to become a devotee of pervertism.

Stimulants of all kinds, morphine, chloral, opium, cocaine and allied drugs are in turn responsible for the existence of untold thousands of perverts. Indeed it is a safe assertion to make that nearly every one of these wretched creatures is a " dope fiend " of some sort or the other. The relation between the vice and the drugs is not hard to understand. That element of our nature which tends to total depravity is only kept in check by our higher will. Drugs of all sorts — including alcohol — rob us of will power and the baser passions thus unloosed rush us headlong to the deeper depths of vice forthwith. Not much stress has been laid upon that almost inconceivable being, the female pervert. But she is a terrible and a numerous fact nevertheless. There are scores of her victims, sick in soul as in body and for the most part very young and very pretty women. And their seducers were almost invariably persons of wealth and prominence socially or professionally.

The sexual pervert, born in the likeness of the Almighty, but who has defaced himself by foul actions until he resembles the neuter horrors of a Dante's Inferno, how can he be cleansed of his impurity and restored to his manhood?

Some specialists have averred that once a pervert always a pervert. But this is an extreme view to take of the case, it would seem. The tendency among the more enlightened physicians of the day is to treat the pervert as one suffering from a mental disorder induced by excesses of some sort or the other. The late Dr. L. MacKenzie of New York, who had an international reputation in connection with such cases used to effect cures by exactly the same means that he used for nervous diseases. Cold baths of all types, much exercise, light meals, sleeping in the open air if possible, and what he called " shock tactics," such as electricity, boxing, fencing, and so forth, constituted his methods of treatment. Ormond F. Waters, M. D., of Toronto, Canada, used precisely the same methods and with success. In other words, both physicians were physical culturists.

The subject of the pervert is, as stated, as repulsive as it is horrifying. Yet it has been touched upon, if only for the one reason that the victim of unnatural desire may be assured that if he wishes to become a man again in body, heart and soul, such a happy result may be achieved if he will but follow that system of treatment which Nature suggests, approves and honors.

## CHAPTER XVIII

# CONSTIPATION AND SEXUAL TROUBLES

### Sluggishness of the Bowels Ruinous to Manly Virility and Physical Powers.

Constipation is the author of a long catalogue of ailments varying from a "touch of the blues" to some of the most serious maladies known to humanity, including sexual troubles. Also is it one of the most common of the ills which afflict the flesh and furnish livelihoods to the doctors. In nine cases out of ten it is caused by laziness or carelessness. It is a standby of the patent medicine man, as the lengthy lists of purgatives, pills and preparations in the advertising columns of the newspapers will attest. The laxative habit which in some cases is as harmful as the morphine habit, is born of it and holds hundreds of thousands of persons in its ruinous grip. As an authority on the subject puts it:

"It is not wonderful that designing and knavish individuals should avail themselves of the indolence of the half-enlightened and physic-consuming class of society; those who, having a mere suspicion of the truth that they occasionally hear from physicians and from partial observation of their own systems, dare not entirely neglect the important functions of the bowels, but console themselves by taking enormous quantities of quack medicines. By the excessive irritation which these medicines cause to the whole nervous system of the bowels they force them to contract and throw off their contents, leaving the whole tract in a partial and eventually in a state of permanent inactivity."

Besides piles, hemorrhoids, prolapsus of the rectum, fistulæ and other disorders, constipation literally poisons the blood and so the latter not only fails to nourish but in addition works harm to and breeds weakness in all parts or organs of the body. Its debilitating influences are especially manifest in the sexual organs to which a plentiful supply of pure blood is a prime necessity. Existing sexual troubles are aggravated by constipation and in the treatment of such troubles the restoration of the bowels to a normal condition is a preliminary of an essential nature.

It is not hard to understand how or why constipation is such a power for evil. At least one quarter of the food we swallow is intended by nature to be evacuated from the system. This refuse part is highly poisonous. Unless it is gotten rid of at frequent and regular intervals what happens? There is no question but that some of it is reabsorbed into the system for, as a writer on the matter has pointed out, there are a sufficient number of absorbents opening into the lower intestine to effect the mischief if the bowels remain long unmoved. The effect of charging the blood with this filth will become immediately apparent through the medium of the lassitude, the fevered tongue, aching head and foul breath of the victim. Later, and if the condition is chronic, the other ills named will develop and fatal disorders are not unlikely to ensue. So that we have a simultaneous exhibition of fever and weakness, the former inciting to unwholesome sexual desire as does alcohol and some drugs, and the latter increasing through the efforts of the enervated organs to satisfy the passion.

Unless the trouble is of long standing the adoption of a satisfactory diet and daily exercises for arousing the bowels to increased activity will prove an effective remedy, but in case it does not, more drastic methods must be used for a time. Do not depend on purgative drugs under any circumstances. The use of them will only make the trouble far more serious in character and render a cure much more difficult to attain.

"In short — for I repeat that it may be remembered — they who would get entirely well of this troublesome complaint (constipation) must learn and obey natural law, and abandon forever all confidence in nostrums or even so-called legitimate medicines. They must have abundant and ever-varying exercise."—*William A. Alcott, M.D.*

Cultivate an appetite for acid fruits, such as oranges, apples, pears, cherries, strawberries, blackberries, etc. Avoid white flour as you would a poison. Many suffer seriously from this ailment simply on account of this one article of diet. Superfine white flour has a most powerful binding influence on the bowels, no matter in what form it may be eaten — bread, biscuit or pastry. Eat whole-wheat bread when you can get it, and, if possible, have all articles of food requiring flour made with whole-wheat flour. Raw flaked grains of wheat, rye or oats is perhaps the most effective food that can be used for exciting the bowels to action.

If you are careful not to eat too fast and not to over-eat, and if you combine acid fruits with the whole-wheat bread or raw flaked grains you will usually find that your trouble will disappear in short order, provided, of course, that you also take the exercises advised with regularity.

If, however, you find that you do not obtain relief, there are more effective means yet that can be adopted to bring about the desired results. The massage or kneading process is of great assistance when all other means fail. Lie on the back. Now put a little sweet oil in the open hands, bring them over the adbomen, rubbing in all directions and pressing down vigorously. After continuing this for from three to five minutes, roll the closed hand back and forth over the abdomen, pressing as before. In this part of the treatment the hand should travel in a circle. Beginning at the lower right hand side, then go upward on the right side, over to upper left side, down left side to lower left side, then over to lower right side. This kneading process, working round and round the abdomen, should be continued from ten to fifteen minutes if the case is at all serious. It should be productive of satisfactory results forthwith, though after waiting a reasonable time, you can then resort to the internal bath treatment; that is, flushing the colon. This will, of course, produce rapid action, but it is well to avoid the use of this means if possible as the bowels should not be taught to depend on artificial means for elimination. It is, however, so much superior and effective than purgatives that there is no comparison. Once more let it be said that purgatives cause serious injury, while this means of evacuating the bowels produces no evil results as far as actual injury to the bowels is concerned. The only objection to the bath is that should its use be continued for a long period, the bowels might lose tone and at length depend upon it to produce action on their part.

## CHAPTER XIX

## CAUSE AND CURE OF PREMATURITY

The Mental Perturbations of the Victims of This Complaint — Caused by Nervous Defects and Cured by a Proper Régime.

In all the long list of sexual troubles to which humanity, through its sins or follies has fallen heir to, there is none more humiliating than that to which we may give the name of prematurity.

Usually the outcome of youthful vices, or the excesses of young manhood, it is always a sign of a weakened and unbalanced nervous system. Its demonstrations take the form of involuntary emissions of semen under the stimulus of anticipated or attempted sexual intercourse. Sometimes such emissions will occur while the sufferer is in conversation with a female companion; in other cases they may be deferred until the very first stages of the act of coition. In any event they are of so premature a nature, that procreation is impossible and shame and disappointment are felt alike by both parties to the attempted union.

It has been said on several occasions in this book that the nervous and the sexual systems are so involved each in each, that anything wrong with the one affects the other also. We see a striking proof of this in this instance. The muscles are controlled by the nerves and the latter are in turn the servants of the mentality or, as one may say, the man himself. But sexual excesses weaken the man throughout. His mentality loses its grip upon his nerves, and his nerves upon his muscles. During the act of sexual intercourse and in the case of a healthy man, emission does not take place until the mentality telegraphs to the nerves that the body's craving for sexual enjoyment has been satisfied up to the point of consummation. Then the nerves actuate the muscles concerned and at the appropriate moment an orgasm ensues.

But with one afflicted with prematurity, the mentality is out of touch with nerves and muscles, or at all events, cannot control them. So that the desire of the mind is followed more or less quickly by the act of the body and the humiliated bridegroom feels the bitterest shame that ever man can know.

In some instances, however, sheer nervousness has induced prematurity in otherwise healthy men. Such cases are not uncommon among the newly married. Time and familiarity with the object of the victim's desire will usually effect a cure, however. But it is well to diet and exercise as here suggested, even if it is felt that the trouble is not the result of any permanent defect of one's system.

Where a man is of a full habit, has

strong sexual desires and takes but little out-of-door exercise, these things are to be condemned; very hearty eating, the excessive use of meats, condiments or stimulating drinks, heavy clothing, hot rooms, and "spicy" conversation. Each and all of them tend to the trouble in question.

It should not be forgotten, too, that prematurity is a malady of a progressive sort. After a time the tendency to incontinence of the seminal fluid becomes more marked and finally emissions begin to take place under very slight provocation indeed. The sufferer is now on his way to impotence, sterility or a general breakdown of his system. This applies more particularly to those whose prematurity is due to indifferent nerve force caused by excesses. Yet the malady, no matter what its root, permits of no trifling. Steps should be taken to check it in its inception lest it reach the chronic stage. No man can afford to tolerate or ignore the tremendous drain on his vitality which is inseparable from involuntary seminal losses.

In treating the trouble it is well to remember that the primary object of such treatment is the attainment of superior nervous force. To repeat, there is something wrong with the nervous system in general or the ailment would not be in evidence at all. It is especially important when dealing with maladies of this character, that the sufferer avoids over-eating, although advice of this character is equally appropriate in the case of pretty nearly every physical trouble. But where the health of the sexual organs is concerned one should rise from every meal feeling that one could easily enjoy much more than has been eaten. Two meals a day are to be insisted upon. Eat your first meal at noon, and the second three or four hours before retiring. Absolute continence is trouble. Your mental attitude must be advised while treating yourself for this one of watchfulness. Every effort must be made to bar out imaginations of an erotic kind. Try to forget sex as nearly as you can. Busy yourself with some active work that takes up your time and attention. As increased nervous power comes back to you by these means you will notice that you are obtaining more and more control over yourself. Do not be discouraged if a radical change for the better is not noticed in a short time. The nerves are slow to respond to treatment. You are effecting a change in the quality of the elements of which they are composed. Remember that you must replace the old cells with new and healthy ones before the improvement in your condition is of a notable nature, and this takes considerable time. Two or three months at least should elapse before such improvement can be looked for. The evil wrought by years of excesses cannot be overcome in a week or so.

Cold water bathing is especially valuable in troubles of this nature. It stimulates the nervous system as a whole while it tends to make the organs themselves more healthy. Cold sitz baths should be taken at least once a day, preceded by a dry friction bath. And last but most important, DO NOT FORGET TO TAKE LONG WALKS AND CULTIVATE A CLOSE AND CONSTANT ACQUAINTANCE WITH FRESH AIR.

## CHAPTER XX

## STERILITY — ITS CAUSE AND CURE

Nervous Weakness Usual Cause — Germs of Life Dead or Paralyzed — Excesses Make a Cure Impossible — Plain Advice as to Methods of Cure.

To a great many people, sterility and impotency are identical terms. As a matter of fact there is a distinction with a great difference between them. It is true that the result of each is the same, viz., inability to procreate, and that the causes which bring them into being are of a similar nature. But beyond that they have nothing in common. A man who is impotent is not necessarily sterile, while it does not follow that he who is sterile must of consequence be impotent.

A definition of impotency has already been given in these pages. Briefly and in a general way it consists of a failure of the supply of seminal fluid, or there may be some injury to, or malformation of, the male sexual organ which prevents the consummation of the act of coition.

But one who is sterile may be possessed of an apparently perfect organ and a fair supply of semen. Nevertheless he is in as bad a case, if not worse, sexually, than is the impotent man. Impotency yields more or less readily to the treatment that the author has suggested for it. Sterility is of a stubborn sort and, as indicative of grave sexual complications, requires a patient and faithful compliance with the rules for its cure which will follow.

What is sterility then? It consists of the absence, the torpidity or the death of the spermatozoa, which are the essential fertilizing element of the male seminal fluid. If a drop of healthy semen be placed under a microscope it will be seen that it consists of a transparent albumen-like substance that swarms with myriads of restless forms looking not unlike tadpoles with slender elongated tails. These are the spermatozoa and the function of these tiny creatures is, in point of importance, second to none in the entire domain of nature. For without them, life of all types would quickly cease to exist.

When copulation between the male and female of any species of animal life takes place, the spermatozoa unite with the ova or " egg " of the female and the latter is thereby fertilized, becoming in due season a perfected animated being. Scientists who have watched the work of the spermatozoa under the microscope, tell us how that they swarm about the ova as if drawn to it by an irresistible impulse and, during their efforts to unite with it, exhibit traits that suggest individual intelligence.

As has been intimated, a variety of causes will produce sterility. Professor S. W. Gross states that in one hundred and seventy-five cases he found that there were forty direct or predisposing causes therefor. Authorities on the subject agree, however, that the vast majority of sterile men are the victims of sexual excesses. Apart from these, the malady may be the outcome of intense mental strain, dyspepsia, diabetes, diseases of the kidneys, injuries to the brain, or spinal cord, lead or arsenic poisoning, constant indulgence in lascivious thoughts, friction of improper clothing, too much horseback riding, persistent toying with women, and so forth. Also — and let the man who is in the hands of quacks or drug-dosing doctors note this — some of the worst cases are the direct results of the use of bromide of potassium, iodide of potassium, nitrate of potassium, morphine, chloral, cannabis indicus, carbonate of soda, mercury, alcohol and other like drugs.

"In an advanced stage of the malady the moral and mental depressions are the most serious features, for the unhappy

sufferer is ashamed to seek relief as he would in ordinary complaints. So he is apt to fall into the hands of those rapacious quacks who hire the services of a venal press to promote their nefarious business by exciting fears and delusive hopes by which victims are to be attracted to their toils to be fleeced without mercy."
—*Albert H. Buck, M.D.*

For all practical purposes, however, we must presume that sterility is due to masturbation, excessive sexual intercourse or that it is a by-product of venereal diseases. Some authorities assert that there are three stages of the malady, each of which is accompanied by involuntary emissions of semen, either during sleep or in waking hours. In the first stage, so these say, there are erections and orgasms. In the secondary and final stages, the sufferer is only conscious of his loss after the emission, there being no coincident erection or pleasurable sensation.

Sometimes these losses are intermittent while in other cases they are constant. In any event and in the earlier stages of their occurrence the spermatozoa lose much of their normal activity and are sluggish if not totally inactive. Still later they give no signs of life whatever and, as the disease progresses, they become less and less in number until they disappear altogether. The man's vital and nervous forces have become so debilitated that he is incapable of begetting within himself these mysterious microscopic creatures, that are the incarnation of every form of vitality. To all intents and purposes he is an un-sexed nonentity.

If such a man be of especially strong physique he may in the early stages of the disease, battle with the drain upon his muscular and nervous systems for months or a year or so. But no man created can hope to achieve recovery unless he determines upon a radical change in his methods of life and the adoption of some system of treatment which shall insure recovery. If he neglects himself, impotence pure and proper is but one of the many evils that is lying in wait for him. It stands to reason that a man deprived of the basic power and principle of his life — the corner-stone of his physical and mental health,— is open to attack from all manner of maladies. Nature takes care that the useless shall not cumber the ground for long. So that the insane asylum or the premature grave is the invariable lot of the sterile man.

Yet the causes which tend to sterility suggest its cure. If we reverse the operation, so to speak, and, instead of doing and thinking those things that fill our minds with evil, our bodies with weakness, our nervous systems with nameless terrors and our organs of generation with dead spermatozoa, we determine that we will live lives that shall make for clean mentalities and strong, pure bodies, we shall become as fruitful in every way as we are now barren.

To bring about this happy result, order your daily life as follows:

Before rising from your bed, take a number of deep, full breaths, expanding the region of the abdomen as much as possible. Before you do this be sure that the windows of your room are wide open, so as to admit plenty of fresh, pure air. Next, and while still in bed, take the exercises for acquiring general nervous vigor, illustrated in this book. Follow with a cold sitz bath. Remain in the bath for from one to two minutes, but never for so long a period that after drying yourself, you do not experience a sensation of comfortable warmth.

Active open air occupation is much preferable to sedentary work but if you are compelled to labor indoors you should spend as much time as possible in taking long walks to the accompaniment of much deep breathing.

Two meals per day are much better than

three meals, although if you are apparently digesting the latter without trouble, there may be no special need for a change. Remember never to eat without an appetite. Every particle of food must be turned into good rich blood, and food eaten without desire or relish makes a poor quality of blood. Eat what you like best but always see to it that it is good, wholesome, nourishing food. Don't stuff at meals and don't nibble between them. Eat your last meal three or four hours before retiring. Before going to sleep it is well to take the same system of exercise as has been recommended for use in the morning, always provided you are not too tired from the exertions of the day.

Never overlook the necessity for pure air. Keep the windows wide open. Take hot baths, once or twice a week, and let them follow your exercises. Don't clothe yourself too heavily either at night or day. Drop excesses of every kind. Throw the contents of your medicine bottles into the sink. Cleanse your mind as well as your body. Be patient, persevere in your exercises and realize that you are on the way to fruitful manhood again.

# CHAPTER XXI

## CAUSES OF IMPOTENCE

### They are Many and of a Varied Character

Impotence may result from any one of a number of conditions that are antagonistic to the well being of the body. Unlike the majority of sexual troubles, a large proportion of cases of impotence are due to causes that have nothing to do with debilitating excesses. It is not meant by this that sexual excess is not in many instances responsible for loss of manhood, but it is a fact nevertheless that any method of thought or action that tends to the decline of the physical powers, tends also to impoverish and destroy the vitality of the individual. For this reason, incipient or total impotence is much more common than is imagined. That its existence is not generally recognized is explained by the fact that the victims of the malady are, for very shame's sake, unwilling to proclaim their humiliation even among friends.

Climatic influences are sometimes productive of impotence. A residence in a tropical country, especially under conditions of hardship, is liable to be disastrous sexually to the white man. Many officers of the British army are, through their services in India, badly affected in the manner in question. A recent *cause cèlebre* in the divorce courts of London hinged on the effects of climate. The wife, a brilliant and wealthy woman, had married an officer who won his honors by years of soldiering in India. She brought suit for annulment of the marriage on the ground of her husband being sexually incapable. The case was decided in her favor. Curious and interesting medical testimony developed during the trial, the bulk of it showing that the virility of the great nations of the earth is mainly due to the temperate zones in which they are located.

But it must not be forgotten that the white man while in the tropics and removed from restraining environments is apt to give a free rein to his passions in general. The late shocking revelations of conditions in the Congo Free State are illustrations of this in point. Unstinted indulgence in lust and liquor, to say nothing of the highly seasoned and fiery dishes consumed by the whites on the plea that it is necessary to keep their livers in action, would bring about some form of impotence in any part of the world. Thus are we apt to blame nature where we alone are the culprits.

Improper diet, it goes without saying, kills sexual vitality for reasons that call for no explanation. Cut off the basic source of every form of strength — nourishing food — and so encourage malnutrition and you are extending a pressing invitation to impotence to visit you and remain with you permanently if it so pleases. Remember this never failing axiom — a body improperly fed is always a body with sexual powers journeying toward impotence. There is no departure from the rule. The manifestations of the decay of manhood may be of a larger or lesser degree, but they are there for all that.

In a subsequent chapter something will be said about sexual defects produced by accidents, occupations or those inherited from birth. Such defects, it is perhaps unnecessary to add, are likely to or actually do produce impotence. The first named class is however far from common owing to anatomical reasons. If you reflect on the positions occupied by the sexual organs of both sexes you will conclude that they are so placed that they are but little likely to be harmed by accident.

As far as the second class is concerned, occupations of a sedentary nature that call for long hours and practically no exercise are harmful in the extreme to the sexual powers. Such in the long run are liable to result in total impotence. Disuse of the muscular system brings about a sluggish circulation and the combination is highly favorable to the development of the malady. Some trades that necessitate the handling of poisonous metals or compounds tend to impotence because of their effects upon the nervous system. The third class also is by no means numerous, but to the contrary.

Malformed organs make the act of intercourse impossible and hence they who are thus afflicted are impotent as far as the other sex is concerned. But in addition they often exhibit true impotency, the external imperfections seeming to be a portion of the internal defects of the organ as a whole.

Stimulants of all kinds breed temporary and, if persisted in to excess, permanent impotence. The explanation thereof is that the final stage of sexual intercourse calls for a concentration of mental and vital energy that the drunkard, having lost control of himself, is unable to bring about, or if at all, only after straining efforts that rack and weaken his powers in general.

"Dope" of all kinds — opium, morphine, chloral, laudanum, and so forth — numb the nerve centres and so prevent consummation. The excessive use of tobacco brings about the same result in the same way.

Perhaps the most remarkable form of impotence is that produced by mental conditions. A young man, for instance, of a highly strung temperament is on the eve of being married. He begins to question his power to do justice to himself and his wife that is to be on his wedding night. His "auto-suggestion" breeds ever increasing doubt of himself and finally there comes the settled conviction that in some way or the other he has become incapable. When the time of test arrives the belief is so profound that he actually is impotent to all intents and purposes. The cure is obviously of a mental sort.

On the other hand, intense desire will defeat itself. Cases have been recorded of individuals who never could overcome their passionate eagerness to the extent of permitting consummation. Temporary impotence is also the outcome of incompatability of temperaments, the mutual indifference that not infrequently accompanies a marriage of "convenience," and so forth.

Excesses of a sexual nature cause impotence by simply wearing out the machinery of the organs and exhausting the fuel which supplies them with motive power. Instances of young men — mere lads — becoming sexual wrecks through masturbation are numerous. One of the many after-results of venereal diseases is loss of manhood. Considering the delicacy of the sexual system and the virulency of the poisons of these diseases this is not to be wondered at. Stricture is often accompanied by impotence.

It will be manifest then that, owing to the many ways in which the crown of manhood may be taken from one, proper precautions should be observed to the end of preventing this, the worst of all losses.

## CHAPTER XXII

## MISTAKES OF THE SO-CALLED IMPOTENT

### Mostly Due to Ignorance of the Root of Loss of Sexual Vitality.

Popular superstitions or erroneous beliefs die hard. And as a rule the less there is to excuse their living the harder they die.

An example of this is to be found in the manner in which the public regards impotence. Ninety-nine persons out of a hundred cherish the fallacy that if a man has lost his vital powers he is " done for," for all time in a sexual sense. " Once impotent, always impotent " is the condensed version of this belief. And nobody seems more ready to accept it than do the sufferers themselves.

That the reverse of this is the truth has

been intimated in the preceding chapter. If a man is suffering from no permanent organic injury and has but a little life and vigor remaining to him, he need not despair. A lamp is by no means useless for all time because it does not burn for want of oil. Renew its supply of oil and it ceases to become impotent in the matter of illumination. So too if we renew the oil of life — its vitality — which can be readily done by the means indicated in this book, the flame of manhood is bound to again lighten the dreary existence of he who believed himself impotent.

Another mistake that is also generally endorsed, is that old age necessarily brings with it total loss of manhood. This belief is perhaps the most deeply rooted of any regarding impotence. It is a fallacy though. True it is that when age is weakening all the faculties and organs, that the sexual powers will suffer together with its fellow powers. But *per contra,* if old age be of the mellow, vigorous sort, there is no physical reason why the man of seventy should not be a father as readily as the man of thirty. In other words it is a question of health not of years. One of the most famous and successful gallants of the time of Napoleon I. was a general in the French army who was fully fourscore when he married a young and beautiful woman, having several children by her.

Again the impotent realize that they made a big blunder in ignoring the danger signals displayed by nature in the early stages of their malady. These signals are sufficiently plain and significant and if heeded will avert the catastrophe that is bound to follow on their being treated with contempt. A disinclination for female society is, in the case of a young man at least, unnatural and suggestive of something radically wrong in his physical and mental makeups. If such a person were wise he would of course take steps forthwith to the end of being restored to his normal self. But the very nature of the conditions behind the disease prompts to lassitude and besides that, all of us are prone to procrastination in matters concerning our healths, and so the day comes when the man that was, finds that he is a man no longer.

If, however, he does take heed of the symptoms, he is very likely to make the mistake of turning to drugs for assistance. Sometimes he goes for these to a practising physician, or, if he be a common or barnyard fool, he will write to and get into the clutches of the I-Cure-Men sharks. The results in a curative way are much about the same in both instances. He will lose some money and perhaps more time in the first case, and he will be plundered and poisoned by the bloodsuckers in the second. But he won't be restored to manhood anyhow. There was never a pill or capsule yet that contained the elements of the powers that he is trying to regain. Tonics at their best are merely stimulants that spur a weak organ or function into temporary activity for which it pays subsequently in the shape of added decrepitude.

Others turn to alcohol for aid. These find themselves in a worse shape than ever for, while their sluggish desire may be more or less aroused, their impaired powers of execution become yet more useless.

Still others, with a glimmering of the truth, endeavor to recuperate through exercise and " generous " diet. Such are to be commended, yet it must be remembered that the relations between food and the muscular system are of a very close sort indeed. Unless the diet is adjusted to the special needs of the body, unless the exercises are proportioned to the power or weakness of the physical system, and unless, too, such exercises call into being those sets of muscles whose re-vitalizing and strengthening is most desirable, much more harm than good may result to the experimenter. A knowledge of anatomy and a thorough understanding of the possibilities of food stuffs are essentials in the evolution of a curative system of a natural sort. To these must be added an acquaintance with physical culture and in particular as applied to the requirements of the impotent. The methods advocated in this book are the outcome of these several things, and they are in harmonic proportion each to each.

The list of the mistakes of those affected in the manner in question might be multiplied indefinitely. But it will be found that each one of them is due to an almost incredible ignorance of nature and her ways. Impotence is always preceded by a " running down " of the system, the predisposing or actual cause of which it is always possible to ascertain. But instead of so doing, the patient treats impotence as a separate trouble, apart from that which produced it—an enfeebled constitution. So he endeavors to destroy the growth by culling the flower, instead of striking at the root itself.

No, believe me, there is only one way of recovering your lost vitality and that is by retracing your steps along the path that led you to your present unhappy condition. You are being punished for ignoring nature; now honor her by observing her precepts as told in this book and see how readily and generously she will aid you.

# CHAPTER XXIII

## TREATMENT OF IMPOTENCE

The Natural Method Certain to Bring About Desired Results — Daily Régime for Cure.

It should be borne in mind that those suffering from troubles of this nature are carrying in their systems a vast number of dead cells. The muscular, nervous and functional powers are handicapped, not to say clogged, because of the presence of these cells. And it will therefore be noticed that the most important part of the régime for bringing back the virility of manhood is that which cleanses the system throughout.

Activity, in the open air day after day, by bringing into play every muscle of the body, is of supreme importance. Long walks to the accompaniment of deep breathing exercises can be especially recommended. When referring to a long walk I do not mean one of two, three, four or five miles. It should be a walk that will last from three to five hours, a walk that will continue until you are fatigued, until you feel that you can thoroughly enjoy a rest. During the time that you devote to walking or an allied exercise every organ of the body is performing its work more freely and fully and new life, new vitality, is being developed in you.

Drive out the dead matter with active exercise, I repeat. If you do not feel inclined to follow any definite régime, then take up some work which will bring into action the entire muscular system. Try farming, gardening, or anything that calls for long continued exertion in the open air.

The systems of exercises given in this book are of special value, but they can be rendered even more so if you add to them such out-door occupations that will keep you busy every day to the point of fatigue.

That there may be no confusion in the minds of those who desire to follow a proper method of treatment of the trouble discussed in this chapter I herewith give a daily régime which, if regularly followed, is bound to bring satisfactory results:

Don't loll in bed. Arise immediately when awake. The longer you lie in bed after awakening, the more disinclined will you be to get up. On rising take the exercises given in this book for building general nervous power.

Follow this with a dry friction bath, using rough towel or soft bristle brushes, and thoroughly arouse the circulatory activity of every portion of the surface of the body. Follow this with a cold bath, using a wet towel or sponge. This cold bath should at first be dispensed with if your recuperative powers are not very good.

Go without breakfast, swallowing a drink of cold water instead. Sometime during the morning, take a long walk, or occupy yourself with interesting out-of-door work that will exercise all the muscles to a mild degree. Acquire the habit of taking deep breathing exercises while you are thus occupied, and in fact, at all times when in the open air.

Take your first meal at eleven or twelve o'clock. Masticate every morsel of food until it is a liquid before you swallow it. If you satisfy your thirst between meals, there should be no desire for liquids while eating. Eat what you like, and what you think will digest most satisfactorily, though it is well to remember that wholesome, nourishing food is by far the best at all times. Remain in the open air, and take a rest of at least half an hour after your first meal. Occupy yourself in any interesting manner during the afternoon. Your second meal should follow your first by about six hours, and should precede your time for retiring by about three or four hours. As a rule your first meal should be the heartiest of the two, though to a certain extent the dictates of your appetite should be followed at both meals.

After having removed your clothes at retiring, take the exercises described and illustrated for building up nervous power. Once or twice a week these exercises should be followed by a hot bath before bed. Thorough ventilation at all times is necessary. The more nearly you can sleep practically out of doors, the better it will be for you. To this end open wide both doors and windows. Oxygen, unpolluted and in abundance, will give you health and increased powers in general.

# CHAPTER XXIV

## UNDEVELOPED OR WASTED ORGANS

Due for the Most Part to Abuse of the Sexual Powers — Cure for Same.

Atrophy or wasting away of any part of the body may be produced by the abuse or disuse of the same. In the case of the sexual organs such a condition is the outcome of excesses but never of continence. On the other hand, if the body as a whole is debilitated, and is becoming more or less atrophied through want of exercise and consequent disuse of its muscles, an imperfect diet or other causes, the sexual organs suffer in common with the other organs, shrivel, shrink, and at length are rendered impotent altogether.

The remedy for the evil is suggested by its contributing causes. Build up the nervous, digestive and muscular forces as advised in this book. Gradually your strength will return, and with it a renewal of vigor and your sexual parts will slowly but surely recover their proportions and powers. The importance of the special exercises and general treatment here given cannot be over-rated for the result of them is the making of blood rich in nutritive elements which is in turn sent to the organs and adjacent muscles, feeding and strengthening them as only it can. Cold bathing and plenty of fresh air that is allowed to come in direct contact with all parts of the body will be found of great value. A cure depends simply on your ability to bring back the nervous and muscular powers through the system of physical culture with which this work deals.

It must be remembered, however, that wasted organs are indications of an extremely serious condition of the body as a whole. In short, the system is so thoroughly "run down" in every way that a recovery cannot be accomplished in short order. A return to vigor and health is a somewhat slow process, but it can be accomplished to a certainty provided that the instructions given are perseveringly observed. The value of the reward which waits on that observance cannot be overestimated.

Undeveloped sexual organs are not common, but they exist in sufficient number nevertheless. The treatment for them is practically the same as that that would be in order in the case of undeveloped muscles in any other part of the body, with perhaps some slight modifications of the same.

One of the mechanical methods of treating organs such as those under consideration is massage with an air pump, which is made for this particular purpose, and which without doubt is of value in some cases. This remedy is, however, somewhat dangerous, and if used to excess may produce serious harm. It should be adopted only as a last resort, and even then should be used with the utmost care in order to avoid any possible chance of injury. The device consists of a glass tube, somewhat larger than the average male organ, which is provided with a vacuum pump, that draws the air out of the tube. As the air becomes exhausted the blood is drawn into the organ, gradually enlarging it and thus developing its latent possibilities in the way of size. The inventor claims that there is absolutely no sexual excitement connected with its operation — that it simply brings more blood to the organ, thus giving it temporary and at length permanent new life and vigor, as does a massage treatment when applied to the body.

In some few cases, where the organ is unnaturally small, or where it has remained in an undeveloped state, this device will be of benefit, though as has been said, it should not be used until all other means have failed.

The danger of over-stimulation of the blood vessels of the organ when using a device of this character is unquestionably great, and for that reason its use should cease when improvement is noted.

Any benefit derived from the use of this instrument, however, will be only transitory if the means here advised for general physical improvement are not closely followed in addition.

The device described will be forwarded by us on receipt of price, $6.00, though remember the writer's warning in reference to its use and the fact that it is of no value at all if the cause is simply depleted physical and nervous power. Even when its use can be recommended it should be used only at long intervals. All letters referring to this matter, address to publishers and mark *personal.*

It would be well to mention, in closing

this chapter, that there are a great many who harbor erroneous conclusions in reference to the requirements in the matter of size of the male sexual organ. The adaptability of the male and female organs is remarkable. Unless there is an enormous difference in size the organs will, in the act of intercourse, adapt themselves to each other. Do not come to the conclusion that you are defective in this way simply because you know of some friends who are larger than you may be. The average male organ when erect measures from five to six inches in length. The size and shape of the normal male organ when at rest can be best studied at an art gallery, where nude male statues are exhibited. Before coming to the conclusion that there is a serious defect in the conformation, it would be well to consult a reliable physician.

## CHAPTER XXV

# WHAT IS VARICOCELE?

### Description of the Disease Together With Some of its Causes.

Varicocele is a very common and, in some cases, painful disease of the veins of the scrotum or " bag " of the male sexual organ, or of the veins of the testicles. Cases of the scrotum being thus affected are far from uncommon, while varicocele of the right testicle is extremely rare. For reasons that are yet more or less of a puzzle to physiologists the left testicle is invariably the object of attack.

Divested of technical terms, varicocele may be described thus: around the spermatic cord, which is a collection of tubes that permits of the passage of the semen between the testicles and the abdominal cavity, are wound veins. One of these connects with the right testicle directly and preserves a fairly straight course thenceon. Another joins the left testicle but at right angles and from the first exhibits curious windings and convolutions. It, the testicle, is in fact, completely netted or laced over by its vein with the exception of a small space at its lower extremity. The intricate arrangement of this blood-vessel seems to render it sensitively responsive to any disturbances of the circulation of the body in general and those that affect the genital functions in particular.

This responsiveness takes the form of congestion of the blood in the veins, such congestion being of different degrees. A partial stagnation of the circulation is manifested in the scrotum in cases of the milder type and the patient suffers a feeling of discomfort rather than of pain. He is conscious of an unpleasant sensation of weight or "dragging down" of the scrotum that, if neglected, grows more annoying day by day. There is sometimes an occasional twinge of a neuralgic sort, but on the whole, the trouble in its preliminary stages is apparently of so insignificant a nature that it is liable to be forgotten amid the hurry and hustle of the day's business.

In severe cases, however, which may develop in a few hours or take years to come to a climax, the agony is intense and unless a proper course of treatment is adopted forthwith, the effect on the sexual organ and its functions is apt to be very grave indeed.

The evils that follow on varicocele are brought about in this way: When, through any one of the causes which will be named later, the vein of the testicle fails to do its work, the supply of blood that the testicle should receive normally is either very much diminished or cut off altogether. At the same time there is a tendency on the part of the vein to harden and contract. This hardening process has caused one stage of the disease to be known by a Greek name signifying a " bunch of worms " for the vein, while in the condition described, does suggest a worm cluster to the touch.

This depriving of the testicle of blood results in its atrophy or wasting away. It has nothing to feed on and so it starves, shrivels and finally becomes an insignificant and useless little globe surrounded by the also dead, knotted and leather-like vein. The neighboring muscles and ligaments suffer in proportion from want of nutriment and become lax and weakened. The result is seen in the sagging down of the scrotum which, in the case of an ideally healthy man, should be globular and sit close to the body. The feeling of weight in the scrotum is referable to the same cause.

The suffering experienced in advanced stages of the disease is the outcome of two things, viz., the efforts of the blood to pass through a closing and hardening channel and again, the tightening of the vein around the testicle.

Varicocele is the outcome of several acts or conditions. Some authorities claim that it may be an inheritance of the child from the father, though this is doubtful. For the most part, however, it is the result of self-abuse in youth or excesses in early life. When the sexual passion is brought into play, the organ demands an excessive supply of blood. Its veins are swollen and taxed to their utmost capacity. If the act of intercourse or of masturbation was repeated only at long intervals, the veins would have a chance to rest and recover from their trying duties. But the unhappy slave of sexual vice knows no discretion. He repeats his body and soul killing indulgence as often as his overtaxed organ will respond. The veins thus constantly surcharged with blood become strained, cannot recuperate and finally mutiny in the manner stated. The left testicle, because of its intricate system of blood vessels or vessel, suffers more in proportion than any other part of the organ and the result is varicocele.

Conditions that affect the circulation for ill, night losses, debility of the bodily powers in general, sometimes a blow in the genitals or a strain, constipation or tight clothing may induce varicocele. The writer knows of a case of a young man who slipped on a piece of banana peel. In falling his legs went apart as if he were trying to do the " splits." The next day he developed an agonizing case of varicocele. Somehow or other he had twisted the upper end of the vein of the testicle and this brought on a veritable if unique case of the disease. The injury prevented the blood from freely circulating through the tortuous windings of the vein.

Venereal diseases are a fruitful cause of the trouble. They provoke it by lowering the tone of the system with resultant poor circulation in general and in the sexual organ in particular. The poisonous injections and other irritant medicines used in some of these diseases together with the toxic elements which they themselves develop, alike have a disastrous effect on the delicate circulatory apparatus of the organ.

Varicocele of some degree or the other is of very frequent occurrence indeed among those who neglected to insure themselves a hearty old age. Here again languid circulation is at the root of the trouble. There is probably also a predisposition to the disease on the score of youthful excesses. In some cases the eggs of vice do not hatch out until late in life.

To very briefly resume, varicocele is the stagnation of the circulation of the veins in and around the scrotum causing the organ to sag and droop (hang low) and giving the veins a distended appearance as is seen in varicose veins of the leg or any art of the bod .

# CHAPTER XXVI

## POPULAR ERRORS CONCERNING VARICOCELE

They are Usually Productive of Harm and are Held Alike by Physicians and the Public.

As is usually the case with a disease of frequent occurrence, a good many erroneous beliefs centre around varicocele in regard to its cause, capacity for harm and cure. The greater portion if not all of such beliefs are productive of evil, for error or ignorance can breed nothing of benefit and much of unhappiness to mankind.

One of these fallacies is that the left testicle should normally hang lower than its neighbor. Also that a " saggy " scrotum is not necessarily indicative of weakness but is natural in the case of a majority of people.

Now this is all wrong. As has been related, the scrotum of a man in perfect health, is a firm sphere devoid of droop or any other token of muscular debility. The reason of its assuming the abnormal shape in question has also been told. It is held up by strong ligaments which, with their associate muscles, are fulfilling their duty as nature intended they should when the scrotum doesn't become elongated.

The next time you have an opportunity of so doing, examine a nude, male classic statue, the product, or its replica, of some studio of Greece when that country, the Mother of Art, was at the height of her power and splendor. The works of her sculptors are the exemplars of ideal art to this day and this not only applies to them as viewed by the eyes of an artist but as seen by an anatomist and physiologist also. Do we find the scraggy, saggy scrotum in the case of these statues? Indeed, no. On the contrary we see the tightly-bunched, firm testicles that with the rest of the form, are suggestive of perfected, magnificent manhood. To reiterate, drooping testicles are almost an infallible sign of sexual muscular weakness together with impending, incipient or advanced varicocele. The moral is of so obvious a nature that it would be an insult to the intelligence of the reader to attempt to point it out in this connection.

Another mistake regarding the disease is that it " doesn't amount to much." You never hear it commented upon in this way by a man who has endured the agony of its acute stage. " He laughs at scars who never felt a wound " however, and the thoughtless one will think otherwise when strangulation of the testicular vein develops in his own or in a friend's case. Varicocele does " amount " although slowly in most instances. It is furthermore usually a progressive disease, one that doesn't run its appointed course and then bid adieu to the patient as do typhoid or smallpox. The reason of its persistence is, without doubt, the unreason or neglect of he whom it attacks. Unless such a person is made to realize the danger of neglect, he continues his series of "good times" or his iniquity of secret sin or the abuse of his body in some other form and manner. And, meantime, varicocele is steadily destroying the testicle until one day the man discovers that he is literally but half a man.

The belief that varicocele can only be cured with the assistance of the surgeon's knife is held by a large proportion of the public and by the majority of the members of the medical profession. Very recently the writer was talking to a physician who, with the assistance of two professional brethren, had just performed an operation for varicocele on an apparently otherwise healthy young man.

"But why not use some other means of

effecting a cure?" the physician was asked.

"There are no other means."

"That's hardly so, is it, doctor?"

The man of medicine smiled in a superior fashion.

"My dear, sir," he replied, "I have been in practice for a number of years. Consequently I know whereof I speak. Varicocele of any stage can only be cured by the use of a ligature."

And he refused to discuss the matter further. Just how the ligature is applied will be told in the following chapter. But if doctors are wanting in wisdom in this manner who shall blame the layman for holding tight his pet errors and mistakes. Varicocele has been, is, and will be for all time, cured by natural and simple means except in a few — a very few — cases of the most advanced type. The writer is no bigot. There are times and seasons where the surgeon may be needed. But none the less there are many, many more times when he is a dangerous superfluity. And he is mostly the latter where varicocele is concerned.

Yet another very popular belief, which is alluded to elsewhere, is, that old age is inevitably accompanied by varicocele or at least, a marked weakness of the muscular powers of the scrotum, which is equivalent to saying the same thing. The patriarchs of Biblical times would have resented the imputation with all the vigor of their vigorous personalities in view of the fact that they seem to have been at their sexual best when they were two or three centuries to the good. But even as it is, there are plenty of modern patriarchs who are prepared to give the lie direct to the fallacy in question. The truth is that sexual health should last as long as life itself. There may in extreme old age be a general slackening of the intensity of all the powers, but this is a very different matter from the passing of the years inevitably producing disease of a specific nature such as varicocele.

It would be well also to note in connection with the erroneous ideas in reference to this trouble, that there are numerous instances where a cure has really been effected, but where the scrotum has not resumed its normal condition. It still sags and hangs low. This mere appearance of disease often ensnares sufferers into the belief that the disease still exists, and they spend a great deal of time and nervous energy in worrying because of this defect. Though it must be admitted that it is certainly advisable to have the scrotum maintain the normal position assumed when one is enjoying perfect health, yet in cases which have been long neglected, and where this unnatural condition has been produced, there is no serious need for worry. It is possible to be in full possession of normal sexual powers where recovery has been made and yet the scrotum has not resumed its firmness and the snug appearance previously described.

Where cases of this kind have appeared, unquestionably caused by past errors, and the tissue has slowly resumed a healthy condition, we would advise that the treatment herein given, cold sitz baths, etc., be followed closely, as well as the exercises, with a view of bringing the scrotum back to its normal condition. If after treatment of two or three months there has been no change and you still seem to enjoy perfect health sexually and in every other way, there is no need to give the matter any further thought. Recovery has been practically brought about, but Nature has not chosen to give the scrotum its former appearance, and you will have to go through life satisfied with a defect in appearance, although your general health will not suffer because of this.

Of course we must admit that past errors must have been of a very serious nature to have caused a trouble of this character, and unquestionably a certain amount of vitality has been sacrificed because of these errors. But all that is past, and there is no need to grieve over that which cannot be remedied. " Crying over spilled milk " never accomplishes anything.

Other instances of the popular misunderstandings regarding varicocele might be multiplied, but enough has been said regarding them to show that they are conceived in ignorance and born in the iniquity of evil consequences.

# CHAPTER XXVII

## CURE OF VARICOCELE

### Natural Method of Treatment Insures Certain and Speedy Recovery.

As varicocele is the result of stagnant circulation in a blood vessel of a testicle, it follows that a restoration of that circulation will insure a cure. This can be accomplished by natural means of a simple nature. But they must be persisted in. Perseverance is an indispensable ingredient of the " Nature " method of healing any form of disease. Alleged ' failures ' of the system will, on inquiry, be invariably found to be due to sheer laziness on the part of the patients. Nature works on unswerving lines. From these she never departs. Those who accuse her of so doing, are suffering from moral or mental vertigo.

It is they, not nature, who are staggering from the path of rule and precedent.

To repeat, then, varicocele can positively be cured with the aid of the exercises and allied instructions given in this book. Doctors may take exception to this statement, but the fact remains, for the very excellent reason that cures have been repeatedly effected by the system here described.

The treatment of varicocele by the average medical practitioner is, by the way, of a very painful and drastic kind. Ligaturing is almost always resorted to. This consists of making an incision in the scrotum so as to expose the vein of the testicle and then passing a ligature of catgut around the upper part of the blood vessel. The effect of this is to cut off the supply of blood from the lower portion of the vein, which is in consequence "killed" or becomes atrophied. The testicle is of course rendered useless by the operation because no part of the body can perform its alloted work unless furnished with its full quota of blood. Under favorable conditions this form of " cure " takes six weeks or more to consummate. Physicians admit that it is one of the most risky of the minor surgical operations. There is, furthermore, the danger of the right testicle being harmed by the added work imposed

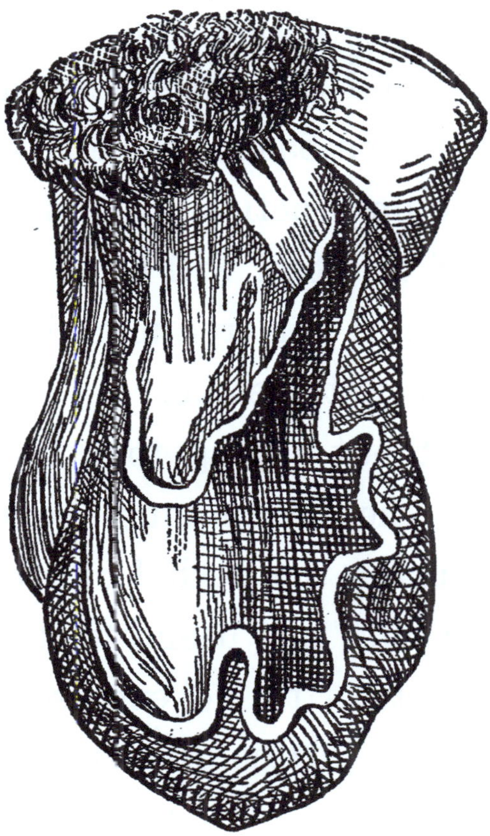

Varicocele and Varicose enlargement of the Veins of the Scrotal Wall.

upon it. It has to do double duty so to speak. Sometimes amputation of a portion of the scrotum is resorted to.

Health and a good, constant circulation are interchangeable terms, or, to be exact, the latter is the outcome of the former. So that the things that make for health, make also for a cure for varicocele. What these things are — diet, ventilation, bathing, exercise and the like — are, as given here, not theories based on beliefs but results founded on practice. A thorough appreciation of this fact will be of benefit to you because faith in a treatment is a factor in the potency of the same.

It goes without saying that the sexual functions of the organ must be entirely suspended during the period of treatment. And, after a cure has been effected, there must be no return to old excesses of any sort. A relapse in this direction is pretty sure to be followed by a reappearance of the malady.

In depending upon nature for a cure, you must thoroughly realize that it is the stagnation of the blood in the parts which has caused your trouble. Now is it not plain that by remedying this fault, by strengthening the tissues and by bringing about a normal condition of the circulation through these parts, that a cure can be easily accomplished?

The most powerful stimulant to the external circulation is unquestionably cold water. In the treatment of varicocele, we attach very great importance to the use of this agency. The cold sitz bath is unquestionably the best method for using cold water in order to bring about the most satisfactory results. In the chapter on bathing you will find a detailed description of the sitz bath, if you do not understand how to take it. This is absolutely necessary to effect a cure by this means, and if you have not a bath tub of this nature you can use an ordinary wash tub or any convenience which will allow you to immerse the hips in water. The duration of this bath depends altogether upon your recuperative powers. If you are fairly full blooded and can re-

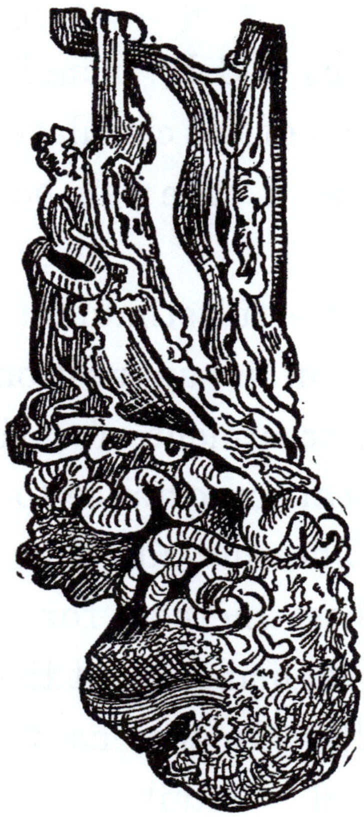

Illustration of an old and dangerous Varicocele.

cuperate quickly with a feeling of warmth, the bath can be continued longer than if the circulation is poor. If the recuperative powers are good, however, it would be much more to your advantage if you remain in the water only one or two minutes, then walk around the room a brief period, and then again take the bath for a similar period. The stimulative qualities are increased by this method. The cold water coming in contact with the skin drives the blood inward and accelerates the action of every external part of the body. The water should be as cold as it can be secured and still allow you to recuperate with a feeling of warmth. If the water is ice cold and you can recuperate satisfactorily, it would be that much more to your advantage.

Exercise is of especial importance in curing troubles of this nature, for as has been mentioned in referring to this disease, one of its principal causes is the general loss of tone in the entire nervous and functional system. Exercise will also have a tendency to accelerate the circulation of all the parts adjoining the scrotum and naturally greatly accelerate the circulation of this organ itself.

Besides the exercises recommended in chapter XXXII we have illustrated an additional exercise that is especially beneficial for those suffering from this trouble. This exercise is recommended because it accelerates the circulation very thoroughly in the region adjoining the affected part.

Long walks in the open air, plenty of deep breathing, can be especially recommended to sufferers of this trouble. A careful reading of the chapter referring to walking will be of benefit as it strongly emphasizes its value.

Diet also is of special importance for the reason that the quality of the blood is not up to the standard or you could not have acquired this trouble. When the functional and nervous systems lose tone the blood always loses in quality. Therefore, the character and quantity of food used is of special importance. Stuffing should not be permitted under any circumstances, the two meal a day plan should be followed at all times, or else if three meals are allowed,

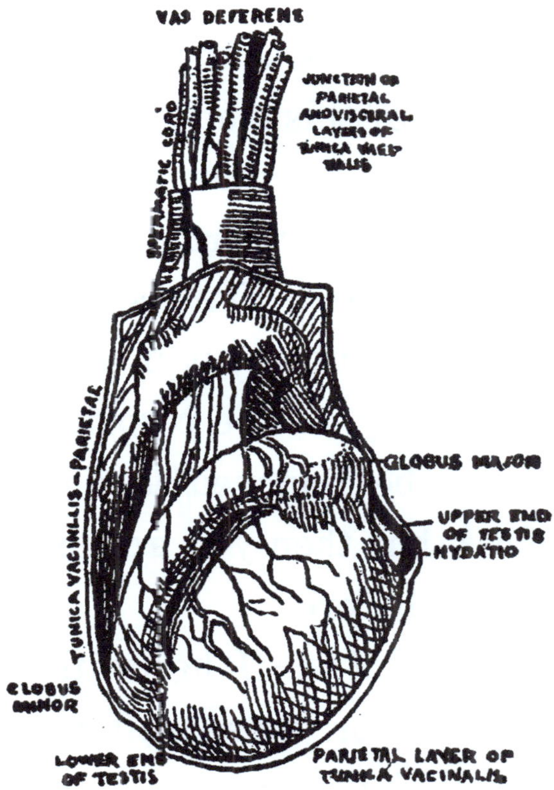


Illustration of Healthy Testicle.

they must be limited in quantity. The cure can certainly be predicted far sooner if two meals per day régime is adopted. There is not only less liability of overeating under these circumstances but the stomach has more chance to rest and can digest more satisfactorily and will make a purer and better grade of blood than when three meals are eaten.

Of course it would be well to remember that in the cure of this trouble we cannot in every case warrant that the distended veins will resume their normal size. There is no power on earth that can cause this result to be brought about in some cases. Of course surgery can be resorted to, and the veins can be removed and made entirely useless, but then you are in a worse condition than before.

DAILY REGIME: I herewith append a daily régime for those suffering from this trouble that they may not forget important parts of the treatment. As the results depend largely upon building up general functional vigor just as does the cure of nearly every complaint referred to in this book, therefore, the régime will naturally be somewhat similar to others advised.

Rise as soon as your desire for sleep has been satisfied. Immediately upon arising

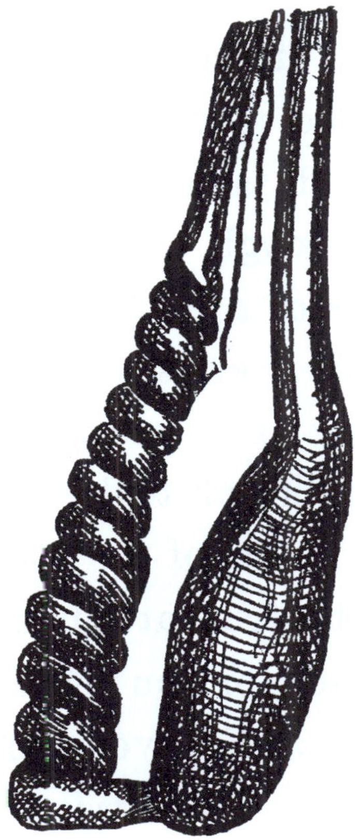

Varicocele Caused by Masturbation.

take the exercises given in Chapter XXXII.

Precede these exercises with the special exercise given in this chapter and follow the exercises with this exercise. Continue each exercise until a feeling of fatigue is induced. Follow this with a dry friction bath, using a rough towel or soft bristle brushes, and giving special attention to the upper parts of the legs and hips. Follow this with a cold sitz bath taken as previously directed, after which dry thoroughly with a rough towel. Don't forget the importance of a long walk with many deep breathing exercises. This is absolutely necessary as an aid to cure.

If you find it difficult to do without breakfast in the beginning of the treatment, you might eat a little fruit at this meal, though it would be better for you if breakfast were omitted entirely. Eat your first meal at eleven or twelve. Have water at hand at all times, and use it freely between meals when thirsty. If you do this, there should be no desire for liquid at meal times. Masticate food to a liquid before swallowing. You should follow your appetite in diet, though be careful to confine yourself to nutritious foods. Pastry, meat, spiced or made dishes should be avoided at all times. If you have a real appetite, there is no need of palate ticklers of any kind. Eat your second meal about six hours after your first, and about three or four hours before retiring. The first meal should be your heartiest.

Sometime during the day you should take a long walk, taking plenty of deep breathing exercises during this walk. If occupied in manual labor, this walk can be omitted, though deep breathing exercises should be taken frequently.

Don't overwork, and don't worry.

Repeat the same exercises in the evening before retiring that has been advised for the morning, following the exercises with a cold sitz bath, though the friction bath should be omitted in the evening. Simply dry the skin thoroughly. Once or twice during the week follow the exercises in the evening with a hot bath.

The veins, if they cannot be reduced to their normal size, will so change their texture and condition that they will be able to properly perform their duties without pain

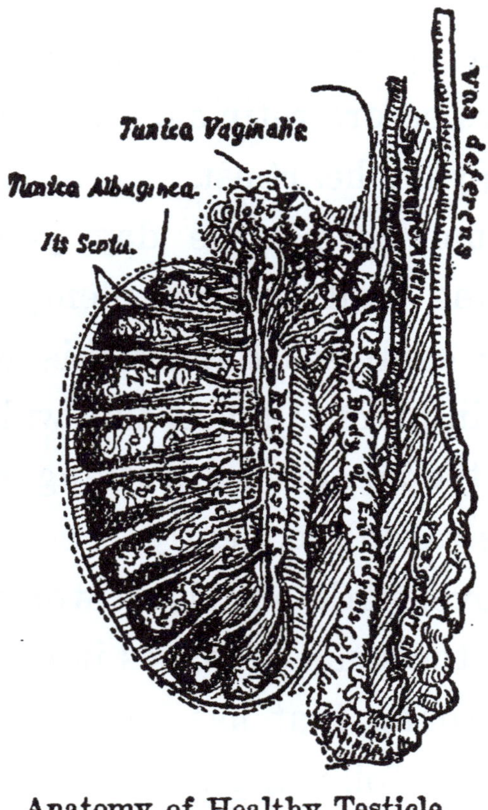


Anatomy of Healthy Testicle.

or inconvenience. The process we advise, that is, of furnishing the tissue with pure blood, not only makes it firmer and stronger, but improves its quality in every way, enabling it to more thoroughly perform its functions, whatever they may be.

In very bad cases the use of a suspensory is advised for a short period in the beginning of treatment. Gradually, however, this " crutch " should be discarded. The tissue can not become strong and self-supporting if it is continually held up in this manner. Slowly, as the tissue increases in strength, begin to lessen the period of time each day during which the suspensory is worn. After several weeks of tapering off in this manner you should finally be able to discard it without inconvenience.

From a standing position bend the knees and assume the crouching position, maintain this position for a short period, then with hands on floor as shown in illustration, lean forward, resting weight on the hands, shoot the legs out to the position shown in next photo.

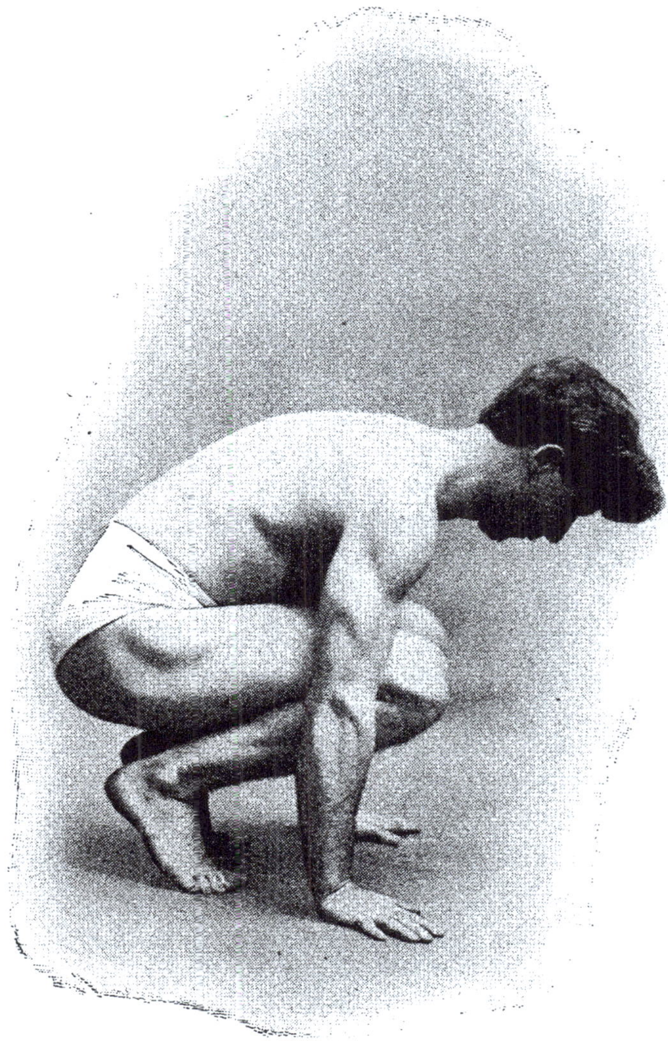

(Face p. 264.)

Maintain this position for a short period, raising and lowering the central portion of the body, then with a jump, bring the legs back to first position again, then come to a standing position. Repeat the entire movement until tired.

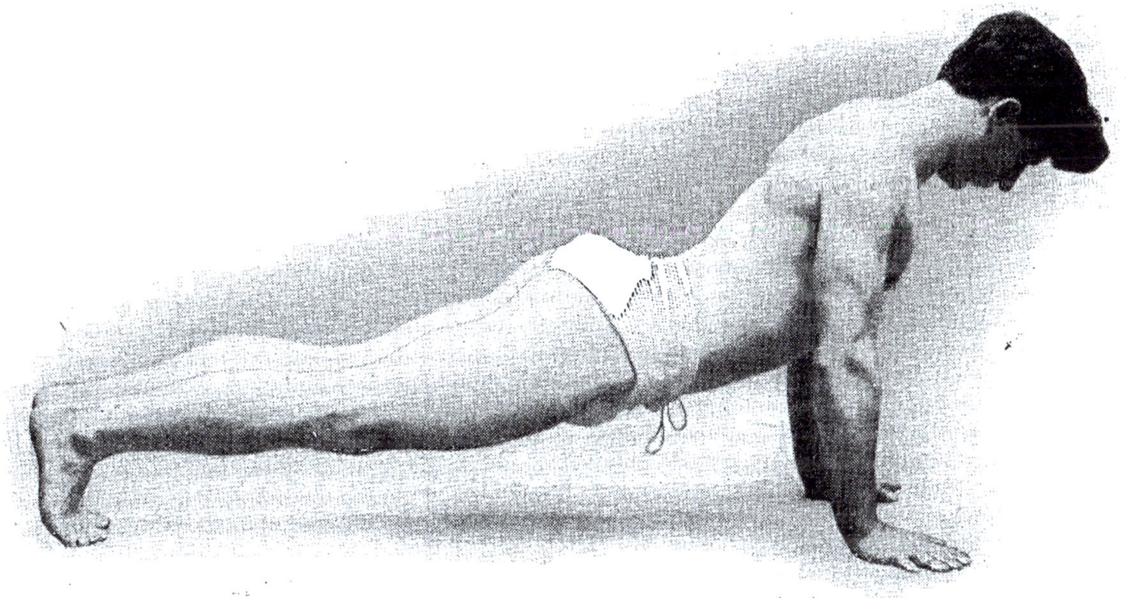

(Face p. 266.)

# CHAPTER XXVIII

## IN BONDS OF SEXUAL SLAVERY

### Every Faculty and Function are Fettered by Unchecked Sensuality.

When a man becomes a captive to sexual passion, he finds that his bonds are metaphorically stronger than the strongest steel. Every impulse of his imagination, every thought of his mentality, every act of his body is hampered by them, and he can only move in the direction or remain in the position that his captor pleases. His subjection is as complete as his servitude degrading. When he realizes his position, if he ever does, he reaps no consolation from the reflection that he willingly surrendered himself to that which is proving to be so tyrannous a taskmaster.

The person who is a slave to drink or tobacco or drugs has only outside influences to contend with. If he can keep away from them, or they be kept from him, he is a saved man. But with lust, it is different. It is begotten in a man, lives in a man, and, until the time of his death or redemption, can be no more disassociated from him than can his hunger or thirst. It is a moral parasite that thrives by the food it feeds on, and, as is the way of parasites, ruins the body on which it has quartered itself.

Then, too, there are some vices that only seem to soil one side of a man's nature, leaving the rest of him clean, or appreciably so. Gamblers, for instance, are traditionally generous and loyal to their friends. The author of "Frenzied Finance" asserts that, away from the glamor of organizing criminal "deals" and mergers and trusts that wreck hundreds of homes and thousands of private fortunes, the men who are responsible for them are ideal citizens in most respects. Our soldiers and sailors are given to picturesque profanity, yet their courage and patriotism are not harmed thereby, and so it goes.

But every atom of the moral nature of the slave of lust seems to be infected with poison distilled by his ruling vice. Such an one is intensely selfish, for he lives for but self-gratification. He is treacherous to the extreme, for a libertine will readily sacrifice the daughter, sister, or wife of his best friend, and what he will do in one he will do in the rest of the affairs of life. He is suspicious because he creates around him an atmosphere of suspicion. He is cowardly for the reason that he preys only on the weak or the needs of the distressed. He is incapable of pure living or high thinking. He is the pole-cat of his species, befouling everything and everybody with which he comes in contact. He has but one use for women, but one thought regarding them. In pursuit of his questionable pleasures he knows not truth or honor, decency or self-respect. He earns the contempt of honest men and the hatred of virtuous women.

Yet, while we may heartily and properly detest such an individual, let us ask ourselves if there were not predisposing causes to his degradation. We must in the first place remember the enormous influence of mind over body, both before and after birth. A man's ability to remain permanently continent depends largely on his inherited mental status. It will be admitted that the average human being of today is born under conditions that tend to aggravate or develop the sexual instinct to an abnormal extent. But few marriages are based on right lines. Excess is the rule in such marriages in nearly every instance, and it is usually continued even during pregnancy at the time that the child is forming and growing, not only in shape and stature but in the way of mental impressions that are to bear fruit in some way during its life that is to be. When this is considered, can one wonder at the premature development of the sexual instinct in children? And with it comes the prudish silence of parents, which to a growing, thinking boy still further arouses his curiosity and his interest. All this combined with the stimulating diet adopted in most homes, results in a boy's attention being further called to the sexual part of his nature, and finally, urged by his prenatal inclinations,— the result of his parents' excesses,— he learns to practice self-abuse, often long before puberty has been reached. In accordance with a well known physiological law, an induced over-activity of one function of the body results in an increased supply of needed material being sent to the organs of that function, but at the expense of the other parts of the body that have to yield a goodly portion of their normal nourishment. So that while the flow of seminal fluid of the masturbator seems to suffer no diminishment, but if anything to increase with each filthy indulgence, the truth is that he is robbing Peter to pay Paul, and in the course of time, Peter will surely discover and terribly resent the drain upon his resources. In other words, there will be a general breakdown of the system.

When the boy is freed from the restraints of home and goes out into life, his now abnormal sexual passion and supply of semen may expend themselves on women rather than in the solitude of his room, but expend they must. There is no middle course. One who has practised self-abuse rarely ever becomes permanently continent. He may manage to escape the clutch of his vice to the extent of revolting at the idea of masturbation, and he may, though not often, indulge his desires only at rare intervals and in a normal fashion, but the seed sown by prenatal influences and in the lusts of youth will, like a poisonous weed, occasionally reappear in spite of all efforts to eradicate it.

We see then that the forging of the fetters of the sexual slave began in the presence of masturbation and that this lust, as has been stated more than once in this book, is to a great extent the outcome of parental stupidity and prudishness. Yet the world grows no wiser by repeated and disastrous lessons. The young man who brings his parents' gray hairs in sorrow to the grave by his seductions, his consorting with fallen women, his evil treatment of his wife, his betrayal of his friends' honor, and his brood of vices hatched by his master vice is, like the poor, always with us. So, too, is the parent who tries to do justice to a child in every way except in that, the most important, of teaching it the duties and responsibilities of its sexuality. And the former is the outcome of the latter. But, except in a very few cases, no voice is heard in protest, no tones of entreaty or warning. The old conditions observe and the old vices remain and flourish.

Vanity of mind or person is a powerful prompter of actions. It is a pity then that he who is in the bonds of sexual slavery cannot see himself as others see him. If he did so his self-esteem might persuade him to that which his conscience cannot. For he is a repulsive looking creature, whether viewed physically or morally, whose looks and form he would assuredly change were they as visible to himself as they are to spectators.

As far as his face is concerned, he appears to be that which he is. His eyes have a suggestive and permanent leer, and not unfrequently there are dark hollows beneath them. His lips, if visible, are sensually curved. There is either a waxy pallor or an unhealthy flush on his cheeks, and the lines on the forehead and from nose-root to mouth-corners are deeply cut.

His form is never good, he usually stoops somewhat, and in time always becomes wabbly about the knees. In business he is unreliable, and socially he is either a cesspool or a bore. The only time that he shows signs of animation or interest is when he is under the stimulus of the society of a woman whom he hopes to get into his clutches. Usually he drinks, for the drain upon his vitality calls for stimulants. Invariably he is unhealthy in some way or the other. He is a good example of those superfluous and noxious things of life that nature removes by letting them hasten their dissolutions by the methods of their lives.

In fact, this feature of the sexual slave is to be commended. As a rule they are not long with us. Sexual slavery causes a terrible drain upon the entire functional and vital systems. But few men have the vitality to continue in its bonds for a very long period. Some have such enormous vitality that they can stand the drain and keep alive and enjoy ordinary health for years, but even in such cases the time always comes when their evil life becomes too much for them, and they either lose their sexual power entirely or else some disease creeps in which greatly lessens their vitality or ends in death.

Nervous diseases of all kinds ultimately attack the sexual slaves. Locomotor ataxia is a common complaint among them. In fact, if a complete list was given of the diseases which in many cases serve the purpose of punishing sexual slaves by destroying their manhood, it would include all the various chronic diseases made possible because of functional weakness.

Now contrast the sexual slave with one who has rightly understood and properly used his sexual powers. Such a man is described by a well known writer thus:

"Where life has been untarnished by the social evil, the sexual impulse marches like a mighty conqueror, arousing and marshaling the mightiest human powers in every department of man's nature. It formulates his purpose, quickens his imagination, and calls into exercise his united powers in the attainment of the world's greatest and grandest achievements in art, in letters, in inventions, in philosophy. It strengthens every faculty, quickens every power."

Truly the sexual slave is like the rooster in the fable: he passes the diamond in order to peck a kernel of corn from off a dung hill!

## CHAPTER XXIX

# FREEING YOURSELF FROM EVIL HABITS

This is Done by Building Up Your Strength of Mind and Body Simultaneously.

Any one of a number of things may open a man's mental eyes to the fact that he is pursuing a career which is ruining him morally and physically. And a recognition of his position is the first step in the direction of his redemption. To free oneself from evil habits one must realize that such habits are evil. As long as the power to do this remains, no one may despair of becoming true where he is now false, pure where he is polluted, strong where he is weak. The mere fact that the distinction between good and evil is still apparent to one's conscience shows that good is yet a part and portion of his personality. A sincere desire to regain the old time vigor of body and cleanliness of heart brings with it the strength of purpose needed to accomplishment.

Sit down and talk it over with yourself, young man,—you who have been having that which knaves and fools call a " good time " for the past few years. Ask yourself what the " good time " amounts to. You work hard at your business or profession and you earn a fairly good salary. Who gets, or has been getting, the bulk of it? The saloon keepers, who tickle your petty vanity by calling you by your first name and, at rare intervals, ask you to have a ten cent cigar " on the house " in return for the ten dollars you have spent over the bar. Try to " hang up the house " when hard times come and see what the friendship of the man behind the bar amounts to. The courtesans who give you in exchange for your cash, questionable pleasure and unquestionable weakness or disease. Test the alleged affection of these " painted spectres of hell," as an English clergyman calls them, when your pocketbook is empty, and note the brutally callous reply that you will be given. The proprietor of the gambling hell who makes you " free of the door " and who serves elaborate dinners and all sorts of drinks without money and without price as long as you can play his fixed roulette wheel or try your luck at his faro table where the dealer deals from a " phony " box, or any other of the games where your chances of winning are about equal to the chances of an icicle in Hades. Try him too, when you are " stone broke " and need car fare. Those boon companions of yours who voted you a good fellow as long as you had the cash and were willing to spend it on them or lend it to them. Turn to these in the days of misfortune and learn the value of such friendships.

You may, if not quite cured of your folly,

try to excuse it by declaring that you have had lots of "fun" nevertheless. Then your ideas of that which constitutes "fun" are vastly different to those of mine. Fun? How about your ruined digestion? What of your shattered nerves? Are you not ashamed to strip and look yourself over in the mirror and note your ridiculous muscular proportions. Do you recollect the array of bottles and syringes and lint, your days of fever and nights of agony? Are you not haunted with the fear that that frightful malady is still lingering in your blood unfitting you for marriage and fitting you for a premature death? Fun? Yes, indeed, but fun that Satan and his imps furnish to the undoing of all that is beautiful and desirable in life.

Young man, there is nothing in it! Recognize that fact and determine with all the strength of your mind and manhood that you are going to shed the old life and put on the new.

As a preliminary to this *renaissance,* this new birth, it must be remembered that the ties and sympathy between flesh and spirit are of the closest and that what affects the one affects the other in precisely the same fashion. Therefore we must have a sound body in which to shelter a sound mind and a vigorous mind to control a vigorous body.

Fortunately for he who has decided to become a MAN once more, to belong to himself and not to his vices, the initial work to that end can be done through his body. A man's muscles are always under his control, but it is a much more difficult matter to direct the movements or impulses of his thoughts. After a time, however, the health and power that are born of a re-invigorated physical system is, in a sense, taken up by or transferred to, the mind. This process once put in operation goes on as long as the muscles supply the stimulation on the lines indicated. Proper exercise is the most industrious and most beneficial of nearly all the hand-maidens of virtue.

One of the head masters of Eton, a famous English public school, had this to say on the subject: "The result of my personal observations extending over a great many years is, that hard exercise in the open air is in nearly every instance an effective remedy against vicious propensities. Such young men who take such exercise make a law unto themselves and pass the period of their youth in temperance and purity till they have realized a position that enables them to marry."

Dr. Arnold, the late famous head master of Rugby, held a precisely similar opinion and the principle has been endorsed by every person without exception who has given the subject attention. Supplement the exercises given in this book with others that may suggest themselves to you, but not to the extent of over fatiguing yourself. Walk to business, for example, instead of riding. Don't forget the cold bath above all things. Be careful to avoid a heating diet or one that taxes your digestive organs. Both produce feverish conditions and fouled blood and these create unhealthy passion. Again I ask that you note carefully that which this book says about building up the system in general.

Proceed to strengthen your mentality at the same time that you are strengthening your physical being. Give the cut direct to your old companions and shun your old haunts. Perhaps you will find this a trifle difficult in the first instance, but it will come easier with the passing of the days that you are now devoting to decency instead of dissipation. A man or woman is not the less entertaining because his or her conversation is clean instead of suggestive. And there is infinitely more satisfaction in a good book or an evening spent among intelligent, pure minded people than there is in loafing in front of a bar or an expensive night in a gambling den. In the first cases you learn and retain something; in the second you learn — evil, and lose something.

Cultivate the society of good books, then cultivate the society of really good men and women, who, by the way, are *never* prigs or bores or hypocrites; cultivate good thoughts, and apart from your exercises go in for wholesome recreations of which there are always plenty.

When lascivious thoughts intrude, as intrude they will, cast them out of your mentality by setting your muscularity in motion. Be sure to observe the rule of getting out of bed on the instant of waking in the morning. Lust is more active then than at night. And when you have become a man again begin to look about you for some wholesome girl who shall share your future. For remember that even when you have regained that which you had lost, you will never taste the true sweetness of life until you become a husband and father. Follow the suggestions given in this book and you need have no fear but that you will be able to do your full duty to yourself, your wife and your children in the dual capacity named. Do not defer marriage until you are in or approaching middle age. "Marriages should take place in the early periods of complete adult life. Children should be produced by the first fresh vigor of parents and anything that exhausts vital force or prevents its freshest exercise is injurious to the race. Customs of society or incorrect opinions which obstruct the unions of men and women in their early vigor, or which impair the happiness of either partner, or prevent the strong and steady growth of the affection arising from such unions, mar the efficiency of parents and are fatal to the highest welfare of the race."—*E. Blackwell, M.D.*

# CHAPTER XXX

## MISCELLANEOUS SEXUAL DEFECTS

### The Majority of These are Due to Accidents, Occupations, or were from Birth.

Apart from the sexual defects already mentioned, there are others that are the outcome of accidents or occupations, or with which their unfortunate possessors have been afflicted from birth.

Of the first named class but little can be said here, and for reasons that will be evident. It is impossible to give general instructions for special cases. Yet the author would advise the sufferer to shun the doctor with the cutting craze — the chap who is never happy unless he has somebody on the operating table, or has a scalpel in one hand and a saw in the other. Surgery should be resorted to only when all other curative means have apparently failed. Of course there are some cases where the need of the knife is apparent to even the layman, but these are happily rare. Nature has placed the sexual organs in such a position that they are admirably protected from harm from the outside. Hence it is that they usually escape injury even when other parts of the body are bruised or mangled.

As illustrative of the point that is sought to be made in this connection may be cited a case which recently came under the personal observation of the writer. A New York longshoreman fell down the hold of a vessel landing on a wooden crate, some splinters from which entered his groin and the upper portion of his sexual organ. He was taken to the hospital, the splinters removed and later he was sent home. A few days afterwards something that resembled a stricture developed. A doctor was called in and declared that the injury had brought about inflammation of the interior walls of the internal tube of the organ, which was equivalent to saying that a stricture really existed and the patient was treated for such. Weeks passed and the sufferer grew no better. Then one day, and very suddenly, the entire organ became much inflamed to the accompaniment of agonizing pain. The doctor diagnosed the development as acute blood poisoning and declared that only amputation would save the man's life. The patient and the patient's wife objected and after much argument the doctor threw up the case in dudgeon. At this juncture an old woman who has an East Side reputation as a "herb doctor," called on the man and took him in hand. She proceeded to starve him, was deaf to his entreaties for whiskey, gave him steam baths with the aid of kettles, and kept the organ constantly fomented with hot cloths and poultices made of leaves of some kind. For some days he lived on a meagre supply of orange juice. At the end of three weeks he was working again. The foulness of his blood which was feeding and increasing the inflammation had been eliminated by fasting, and the local poisoning had been drawn out of the perspiring pores whose activities in this respect had been vastly increased by the fomentations and steam baths. In other words the " herb doctor " had unknowingly but successfully put into practice the curative principles advocated in this work.

Diseases or affections of some of the glandular parts of the sexual organ are not uncommon among men who are constantly in the saddle. Cavalrymen are great sufferers in this respect in spite of the fact that repeated attempts have been made to construct saddles that shall obviate the evil. Cowboys and plainsmen are liable to injuries of the testicles and related parts through the antics of bucking bronchos. Rupture is exceedingly frequent among them from the same cause. One of the most generally used constituents of hair tonics is an irritant poison which acts directly on the genitals, producing inflammation of the bladder and adjacent canals, and inducing unnatural desire, fever, hemorrhage, and, if persisted in, impotence. It is absorbed into the system by being handled. Paralysis of the nerves of the organ sometimes manifests itself among the workmen in lead factories. These are but a few instances in which certain occupations are identified with sexual defects of some sort or the other.

Among those sexual imperfections that are found at birth, is that not uncommon condition of the foreskin which necessitates circumcision. In a few male children the orifice is found to be under instead of at the head of the penis. This is a painful, and it goes without saying, incurable defect. Instances have also been known where imperfections of the muscular system of the organ caused it to assume a curved form when in a state of erection.

Treatment to the end of strengthening and rendering supple the affected muscles has been of benefit in some such cases.

Organs that are abnormally large or small are more or less frequent. In the latter case, the appropriate treatment has already been given in this book. There are authenticated instances of men having been born eunuchs, and contrarywise. In the Museum of the Royal College of Surgeons, London, there is an example where the testicles are perfect, but the rest of the organ is missing.

Curious misbeliefs exist regarding hermaphrodites, of which, for their own and humanity's sake, there are but too many. These poor creatures never have a duality of the organs of the sexes even in an imperfect degree, the popular belief to the contrary. They are always either men or women whose organs are so misshapen or so indifferently developed, that it is at times difficult, though never impossible to decide their sex. Of course these defects are of the incurable class.

The partial or entire failure of the organ to fulfill its functions through mental causes, or to be unduly excited by the same, are as countless as they are varied and as extraordinary as both. But they cannot be called organic defects and so will not be treated of here. In dismissing the subject, however, let it be said that parents cannot be too careful in protecting their male children from suggestions or acts, that, innocent in themselves, may lead to the gravest consequences as far as the little one is concerned.

Women suffer greatly from sexual defects on the foregoing lines but in modified forms thereof. The treatment of these is a science in itself so to speak, although all or most of them are amenable to the natural method of cure. Many of such defects are directly traceable to the corsets worn by the mothers of the sufferers during pregnancy, or by themselves. The testimony of the bulk of medical men is to that effect. And it need hardly be added that these defects poison the marriage bed and murder married happiness.

"Perhaps it is not putting it too strongly when we say that one-third of the great mass of young women are unqualified ever to become wives or mothers, because of false education and inherited or acquired infirmities. From one half to two-thirds of all our married women suffer from some form of womb-trouble. Young girls, who are wholly ignorant of the delicate texture of their sexual organism, and without dreaming of the serious consequences which are to follow, contract their waists, and thus crowd the contents of the entire abdominal cavity below what is a natural position. By this means the womb is forced out of its designated place, and when the strain is continued, irritation and weakness result in a chronic condition, which quickly develops after marriage into the very prevalent 'falling of the womb,' causing a dragging or bearing-down sensation in the lower part of the abdomen, pain in the back, numbness of the lower limbs, and a general discomfort and misery, which must often be shared for years by all who dwell under the same roof with its unfortunately afflicted, unhappy, victim.

"To a woman thus afflicted life is a burden, and marriage a curse, rather than a blessing. False ideas of form, cruel and destructive fashion and pernicious education, accomplish this terrible ruin of human life and human happiness. Cure, or even alleviation of discomfort and suffering, are doubtful and difficult, and the man who marries a woman with a compressed waist may reasonably expect a sufficient inheritance of misery to last all the rest of his natural life. The man who marries such a woman, instead of obtaining a helpmate, imposes upon himself a burden. He may be ignorant of it at the time, but he will be sure to know it later on."—*Sylvanus Stall, D.D.*

# CHAPTER XXXI

## BUILDING OF SEXUAL POWER

### Synopsis of the Methods of Regaining and Retaining Manly Vigor.

Muscular exercises founded on a knowledge of anatomy and physiology and adopted only after a series of practical tests have been made in regard to the specific usefulness of each, can be relied upon to repeat in the many, the results that they have brought about in the one. Herein lies the value of the exercises of which a description will be given later. They are not the outcome of theory or "information and belief." They are rather, the fruits of the things already cited and they have successfully and for many years undergone the severest ordeals to which a course of exercises could be subjected for the purpose of proving their worth and practicability. They have aided in demonstrating the ability of physical culture — of which they form an integral part — to bring about not only an ideal degree of physical health in general, but of sexual health in particular. In conjunction with a proper diet, cleanliness, and good ventilation they can be relied on to do all that is claimed for them and even more. Those who suffer from sexual weakness in particular will find in this form of training the only safe means of cure. As the muscles develop, the digestive power increases, the circulation improves, the nerves are strengthened, and the mind becomes conscious of a sense of renewed confidence. This building up of physical strength affects beneficially every atom of the body. It is of great value to those who are tormented with a real or apparent excess of sexual life. This last is a disease just as is want of virility. But the surplus fluid and the abnormal energy which is responsible for it can be absorbed and used to advantage if expended in muscular exercise. Not only does the muscle and nerve power increase, and the general health vastly improve when this method is followed, but the unnatural strength of the desire disappears, and in its stead there is created a sane, safe strength of mind and body.

Activity is the law of life. Inactivity brings decay. Long-continued stagnation means death. Some men have the incomprehensible stupidity to think that their muscular system can remain idle indefinitely without losing in the slightest that symmetry and strength that it acquired by extreme activity in early life. They seem to forget that a disused muscle degenerates, grows smaller and weaker and is at length more or less atrophied. The lesson so plainly taught by the wasting away of an unused muscle when a bone has been broken and the limb done up in splints or plaster-of-Paris should not be forgotten. Examine the muscles of a broken arm after the latter has had a complete rest of a few weeks. You will find them wasted to almost nothing. There is no more startling example of results of muscular inactivity than this. The entire muscular system will waste away in a similar manner if it does not receive its quota of requisite exercise. But it is not only this muscular wasting process that is to be deplored — the general vigor of the body suffers to a serious extent also. The nervous organism too is weakened in the same proportion, and with this last comes the decay of the sexual powers.

To be sure, if you are leading an inactive life, you may not notice this atrophic process, for if the digestive powers are fairly good as the muscles disappear fatty tissue will in a great measure replace them. Thus externally you may see but little change in yourself, though there will be a tremendous change for the worse in your system as a whole. It may even be that for a brief period your strength may seem almost as great as ever, but when continuous efforts even for a short time are required, the loss of muscular power is but too evident.

Let the writer solemnly emphasize the fact that impotence ultimately follows long-continued muscular inactivity. This is as certain as sunrise and sunset. It is the law of Nature that it should be so. The sexual powers of man were given to him for the perpetuation of his kind. When his physique so declines that he becomes a mockery of a man who has nothing worth transmitting to posterity, just Nature interferes, takes from him his powers of reproduction and often his sexual desire is removed also. Utility is the law of the universe. It is a positive law of Nature that when anything or any individual ceases to be useful, it and its future disappears from off the face of the earth unless steps are taken to reinstate it in its place in the scheme of creation.

The effect of cultivating sexual vigor by building up the muscular and vital powers of the body can hardly be given sufficient justice. If all powers of the kind named seem lost, or if they have so diminished that the intense activities of vigorous pulsating youth have disappeared, they can be entirely regained by natural processes assisted by the muscular movements to be described; since the bringing of rich blood in copious quantities to every part of the body, which among other benefits results from these exercises, is one of the salient features in the regaining of sexual powers. Under the influence of proper exercise for every muscle of the body, the heart with strong and accelerated pulsations, forces the purified blood with increased power through the arteries and veins and capillaries, drives the impurities out through the purifying organs, the lungs, skin and kidneys, and causes every part and function of the body to be rejuvenated and strengthened.

The effects of exercise can be fitly compared to those of a bath. It cleanses the internal system just as thoroughly, if not in the same manner, as hot water and soap cleanses the external. The vast nervous organism, with branches reaching to and throughout the minutest parts of the body, feels the great benefit of this internal cleansing almost immediately. As the muscles grow stronger, firmer and more symmetrical, the power and delicacy of the nervous system increase in proportion; like a violin string that is toned up to the right pitch, each nerve will respond to the harmony of the music of life. No cigar smoker or whiskey drinker ever tasted anything that resembled the full joy, the marvelous intensity and power, of complete sexual strength. Benumbed nerves cannot feel, perverted emotions cannot produce that which is completely satisfying. Something is always wanting, and the one completely satisfying thing of this existence is the throbbing vitality that is born of the fruition of physical strength which in turn is the outcome of proper exercise.

# CHAPTER XXXII

## GENERAL EXERCISES FOR DEVELOPING SEXUAL VIGOR

These Increase Vitality and Bring All the Muscles of the Central Portions of the Body into Healthful Action.

The exercises given in this chapter are specially applicable to all troubles where the organs of sex need special stimulation. They should not be used when suffering from ailments in which the organs of sex are already over-stimulated. Those suffering from masturbation, spermatorrhea, night losses, or prematurity, should take those exercises given in following chapter and avoid those given in this chapter.

Any system of exercise that brings into use to a moderate degree any of the muscles of the body will be found beneficial in accelerating the circulation and increasing some if not all the physical powers of man; but those movements that are especially adapted to strengthening the muscles of those parts of the body surrounding or intimately connected with the organs of sex will be found much more valuable than the unspecialized exercises by speedily producing the desired results. The exercise of these muscles accelerates the nutrition and strengthens parts, through the working of a well known physiological law which is to the effect that nature gives a copious supply of blood to muscles that are in action, while she makes no special effort on behalf of those that are at rest. So the working muscles are well fed while the lazy ones are comparatively starved; and naturally the benefit which accrues to them, by the renewed life brought by the quickened circulation, is shared by the sexual organs also. Thus, in selecting a system of muscular exercise especially for strengthening and for bringing into being dormant sexual powers, the writer has devised a series of movements that strengthen not only the lungs, heart and organs of digestion and general vital system, but directly affect the sexual organs by vastly increasing the supply of blood to all the surrounding parts.

The amount of exercise that should be taken by each individual at the start must be determined by the strength possessed by him. Continue each movement until a slight feeling of fatigue ensues. Rest a moment only, and then pass on to the next exercise. Be very careful not to exert yourself too much at first.

In commencing the course take each movement say five or eight times. Increase by one or two each day, and after having practiced daily for ten days or two weeks, each exercise can then be continued until you feel really tired.

The exercise should be taken while lying in bed, and immediately on awakening.

Your room should, of course, be thoroughly supplied with fresh air by proper ventilation at all times, but especial care must be taken to insure a plentiful supply of pure air when taking these exercises.

When thoroughly awake throw the covers off and open the windows wide. If especially cold, a few of the exercises can be taken to warm the body, before throwing off the bedding, though it will be found of advantage for you to accustom yourself gradually to cold air. But there is no need of exposing yourself too much in the first instance.

A safe rule in exercise as in most things of life is to be very moderate in any change you intend to make. Do not go in for too radical a departure from your usual old ways when you are adopting new ones.

As soon as you are inured to the cold air, instead of merely throwing off the covers, you should, in addition, remove every particle of clothing, so that you can take your exercise entirely nude, but do not try this at first.

The writer repeats: *Be Moderate!* Feel your way, step by step!

When a man sees and feels that he can practically be born over again, that he can be made almost like a new being by a systematic physical culture régime, if there is a spark of vitality within him, he will immediately endeavor to secure the rewards so easily within his reach.

If you have had the usual experience of devitalized men you have no doubt spent large sums of money and still larger quantities of time in searching for the remedy that we offer you in this book for practically nothing. Give the methods here advised a trial for two weeks, and after that there will be no need to spur you on to further efforts — you will continue on in the good work without the necessity of any incentives.

If you feel tired before going through

the movements to be described, do not try to accomplish them all the first few times. At the conclusion of your reclining exercises, stand on the floor and take an exercise similar to jumping a rope until you begin to breathe freely, then draw in a few deep inhalations, after which take a cold sitz bath as has been told. If this cannot be done conveniently, have a cold sponge bath, not forgetting to allow spongefuls of cold water to run freely over the private organs.

After the bed covers are removed you can begin the exercises, bearing in mind the instructions given in reference to how long each movement should be continued.

*Exercise No. 1.*—Recline flat on back, raise the hips as high as you can off the bed, the weight, of course, resting on heels and back between shoulders. For muscles on posterior portion of hips and small of back.

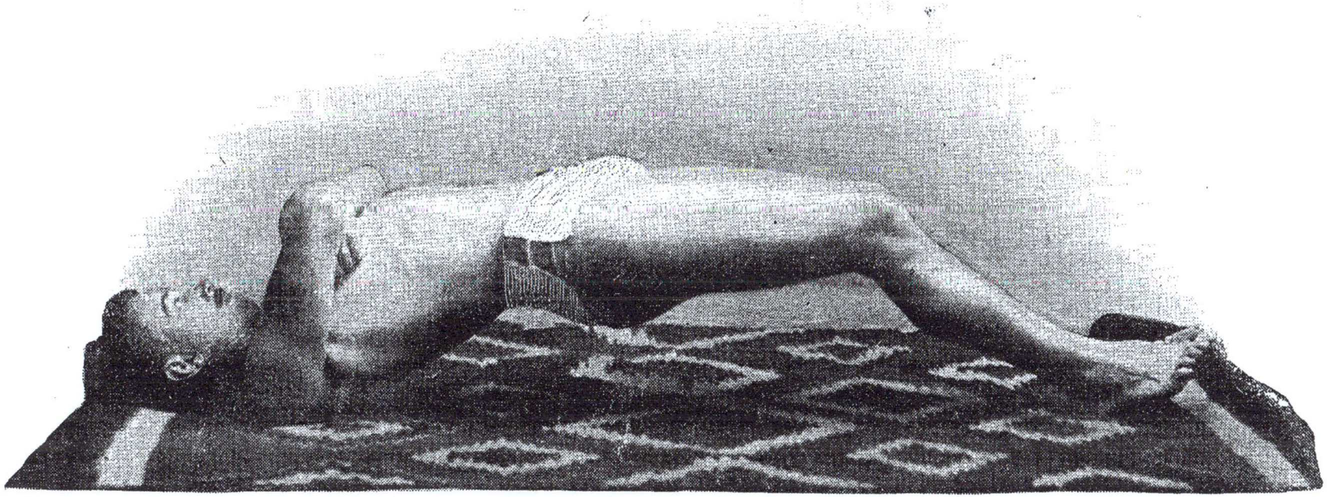

Exercise No. 1.

*Exercise No. 2.*—Recline on right side. Now raise the hips (knees straight) as high as possible from the bed, the weight resting on right foot and right arm and shoulder. The same exercise reclining on the left side. For muscles on sides from waist to thighs.

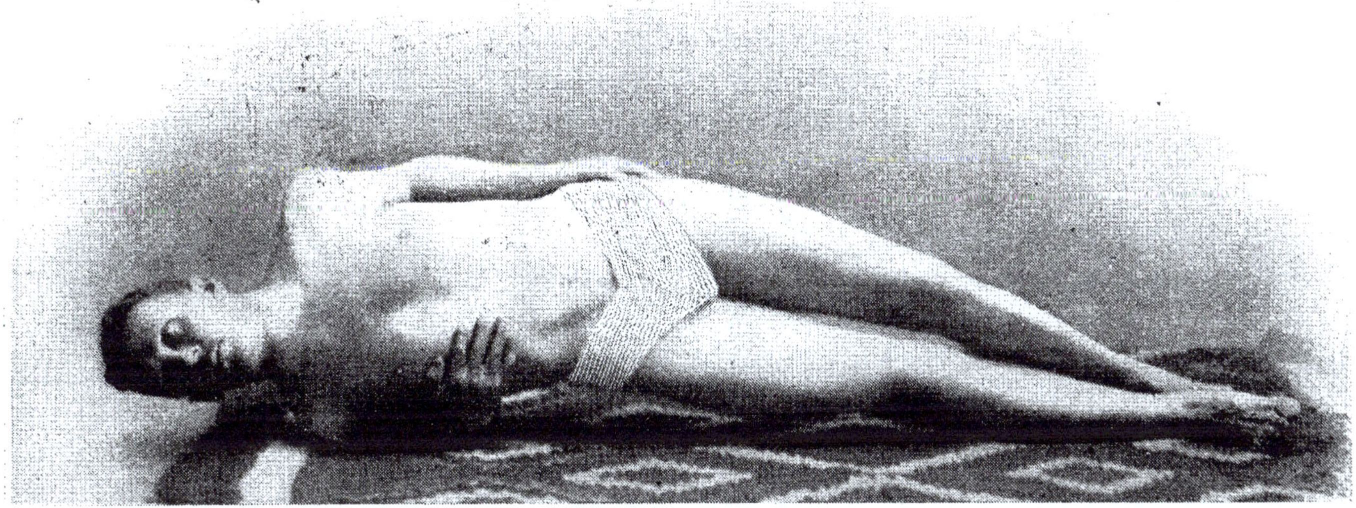

Exercise No. 2.

*Exercise No. 3.*—Recline on the back and place some covers over the feet to hold them down. Now, with hands placed on thighs, raise to a sitting position without assistance from the hands. For the muscles of the abdomen.

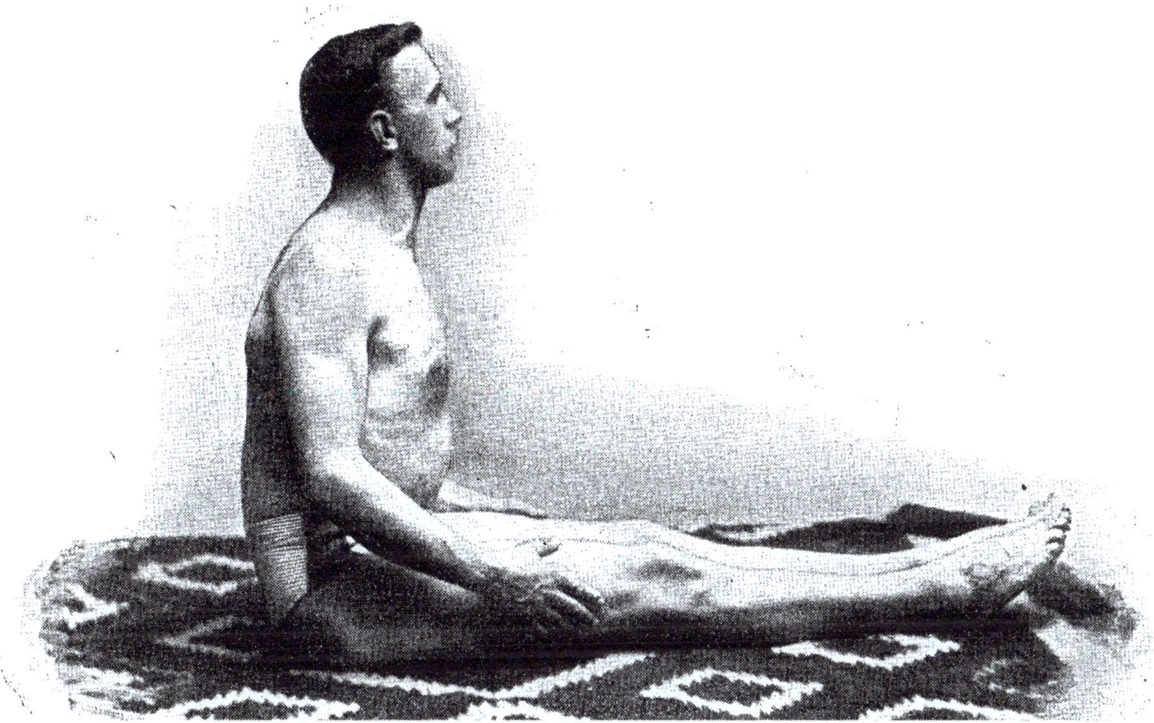

Exercise No. 3.

*Exercise No. 4.*—Recline on the stomach. Grasp the head of the bed tightly with the hands. Next, without bending the knees, raise both legs as high as you can. Not very much of a movement can be made in this exercise, but it is valuable for strengthening the muscles of small of back, and large muscles on posterior portion of hips.

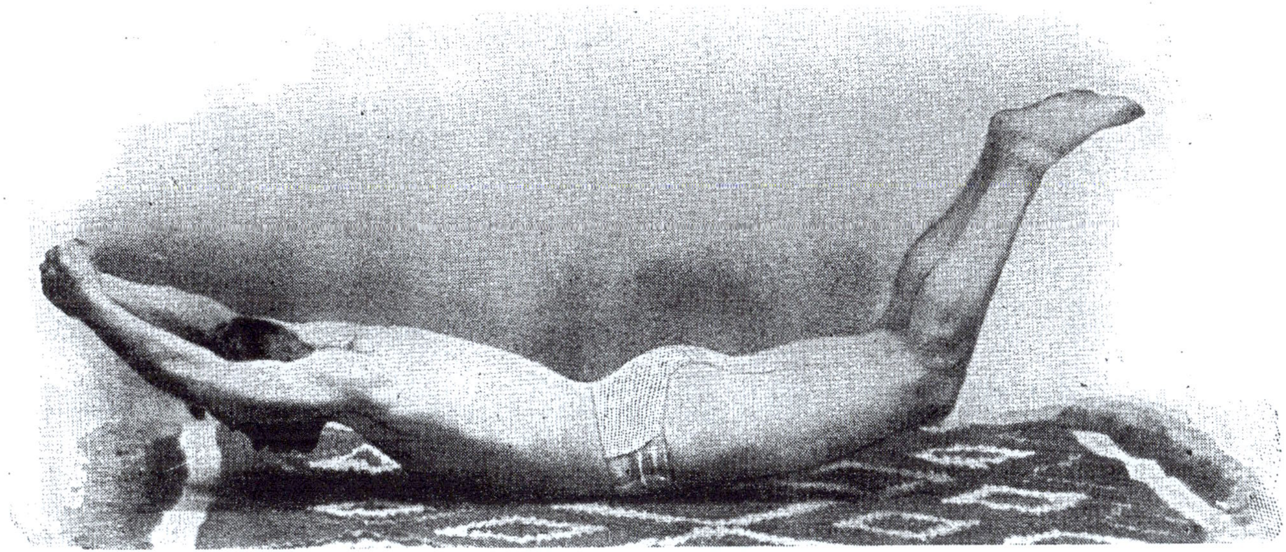

Exercise No. 4.

*Exercise No. 5.*—Recline on back. Raise right leg with knee straight until as illustrated. Same exercise with left leg. For muscles of anterior portion of upper thighs.

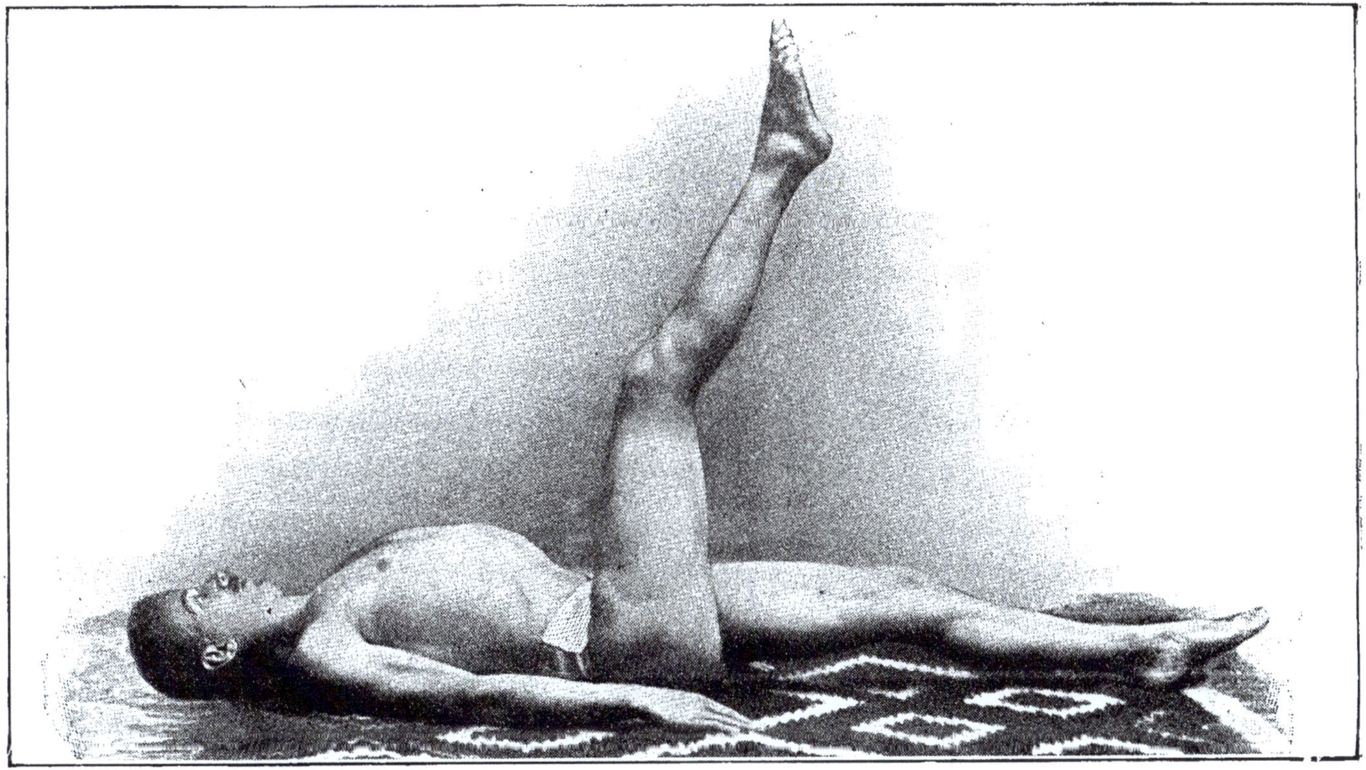

Exercise No. 5.

*Exercise No. 6.*—Recline on right side. Slowly raise left leg with knee straight as high as you can upward. Same exercise with right leg while reclining on left side. For outer portion of upper thighs.

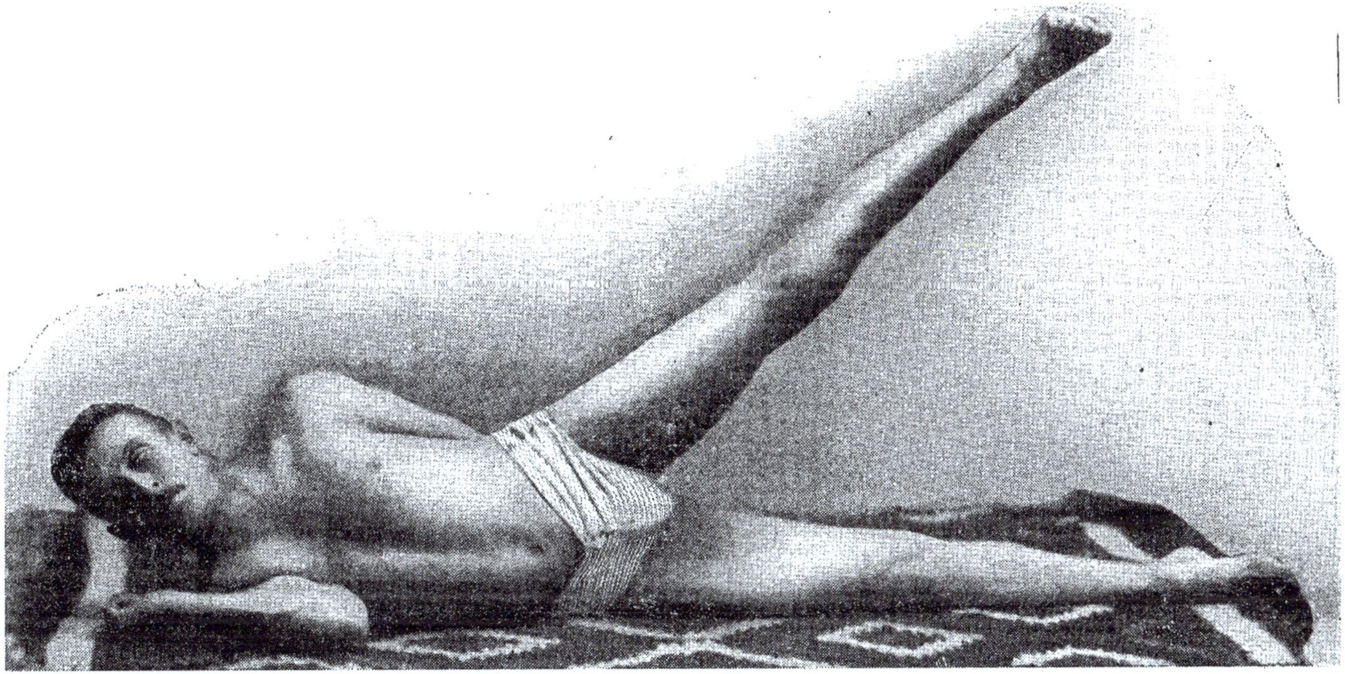

Exercise No. 6.

*Exercise No. 7.*—Recline on back. Then bring right leg with knee straight as far as possible over left leg. Same exercise with left leg. For muscles on inside of upper thighs.

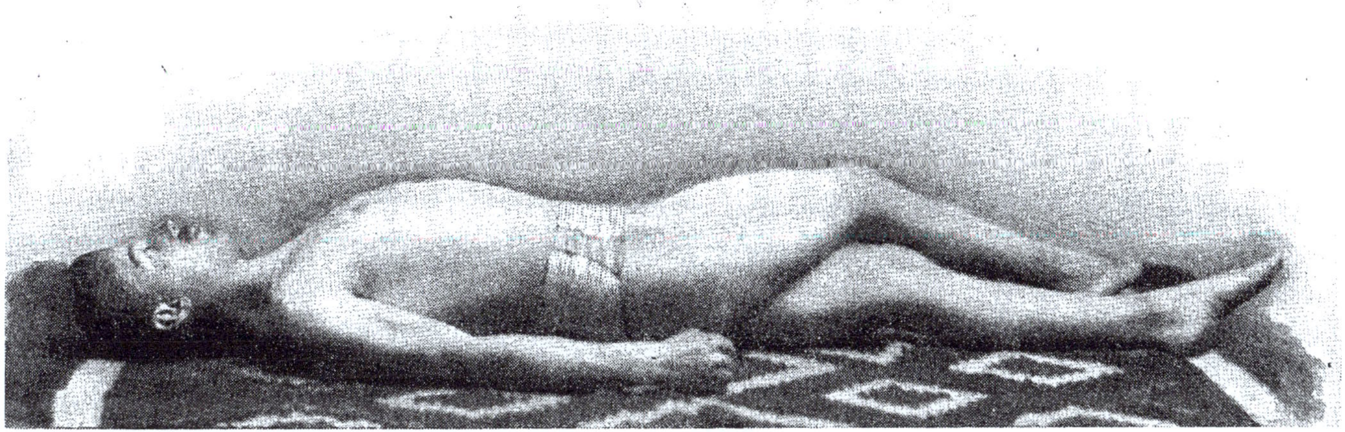

Exercise No. 7.

*Exercise No. 8.*—Recline on stomach. Now raise right leg with knee straight as far upward as possible. Same exercise with left leg. For muscles on posterior portion of hips.

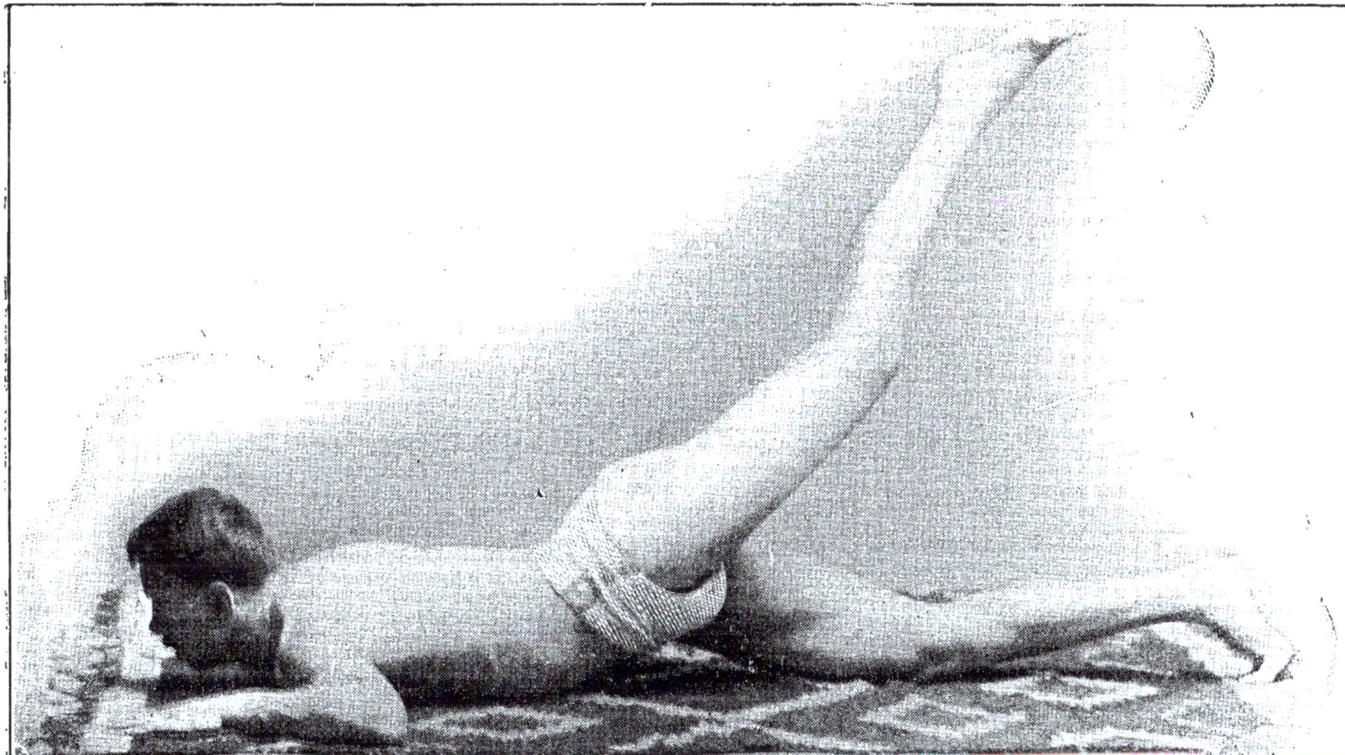

Exercise No. 8.

*Exercise No. 9.*—Recline on back. Now grasp hold of something behind the head, then raise both feet as high as you can. For muscles of lower part of abdomen and upper part of thighs.

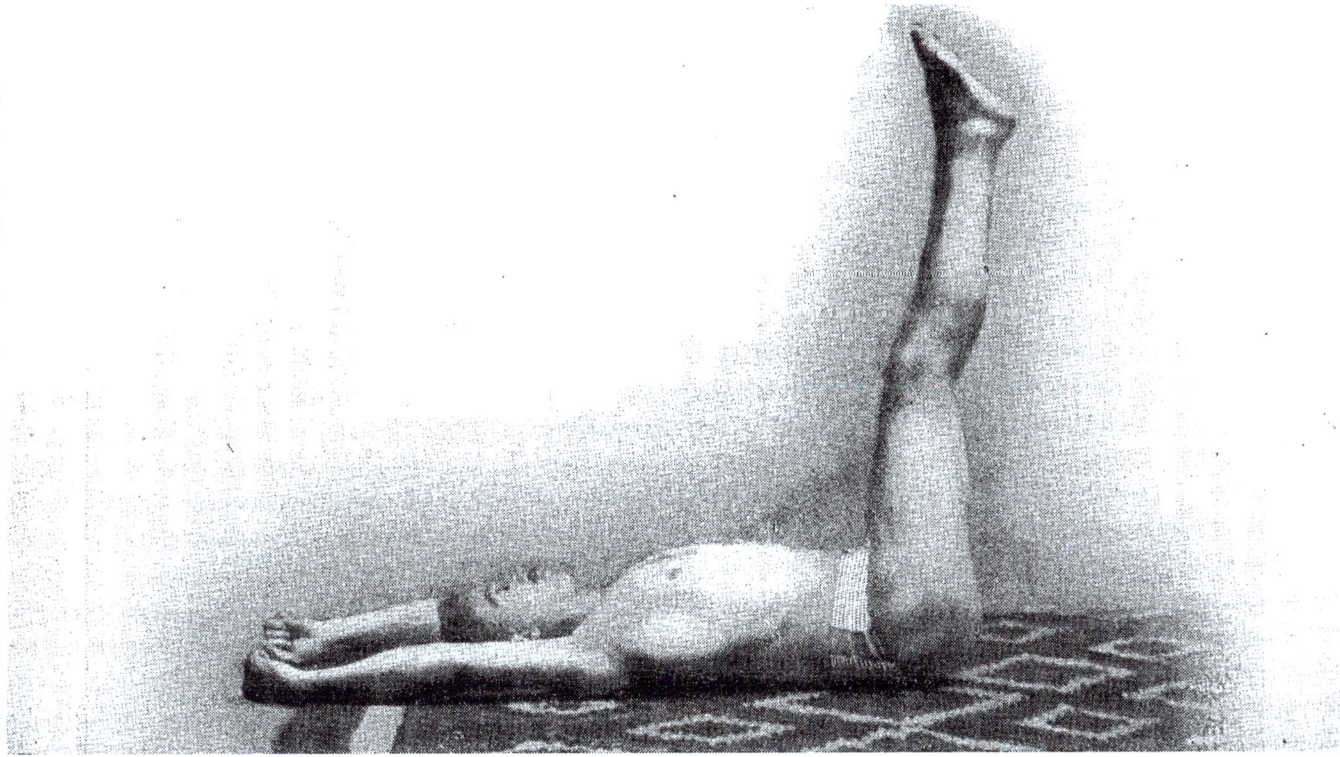

Exercise No. 9.

*Exercise No. 10.*—Recline on back. Bend both your knees as much as possible, and kick out straight upward with right and left legs alternately. For muscles in central portion of upper leg.

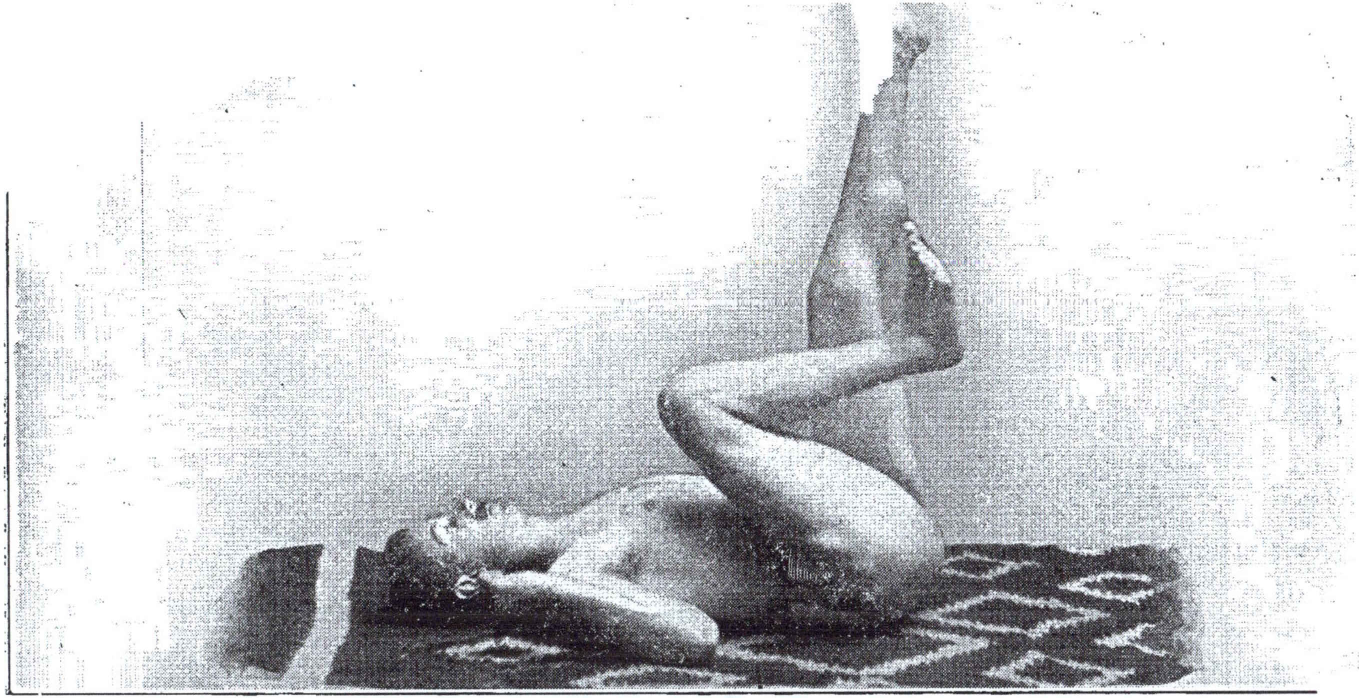

Exercise No. 10.

*Exercise No. 11.*—Recline on right side. Cross the right leg at ankle over left leg just above knee, then raise the hips as high as you can, the weight resting on right shoulder and left leg. Same exercise reclining on left side. For muscles on inside of thighs and lateral portion of waist.

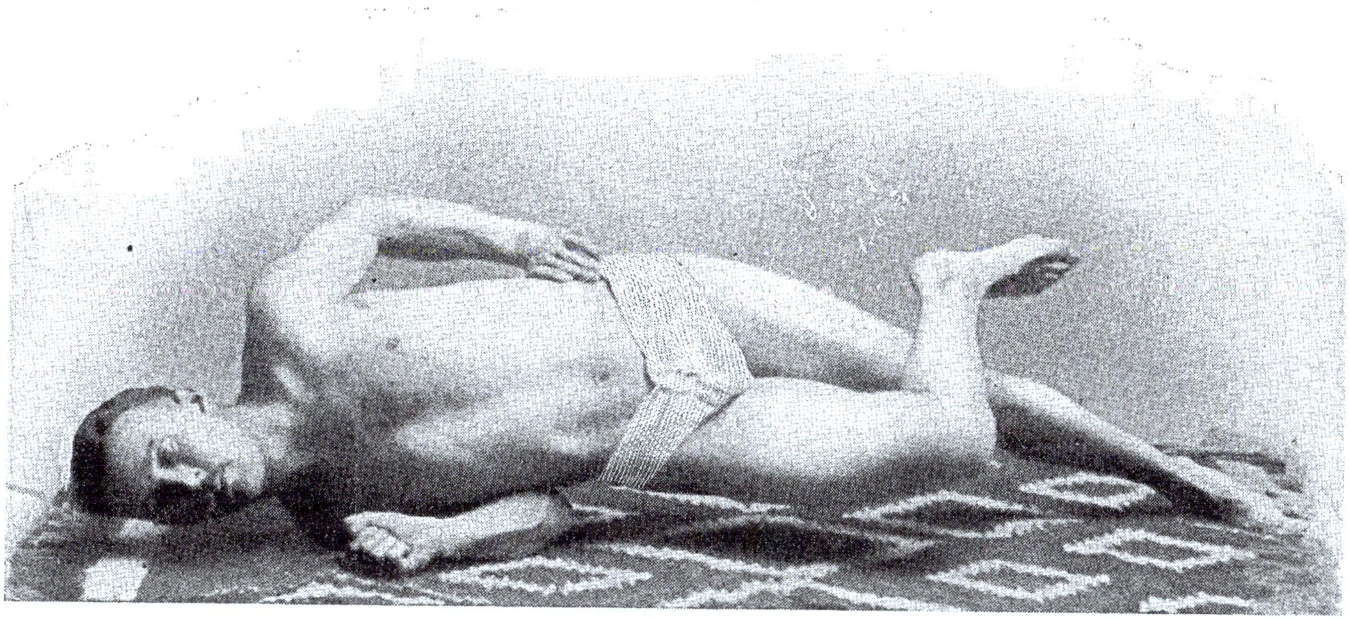

Exercise No. 11.

*Exercise No. 12.*—Recline on stomach. Now cross the right ankle over the left ankle, then bend the left leg at knee as much as possible, raising the weight of lower right leg. Same exercise with right leg. For muscles of the posterior portion of central upper leg.

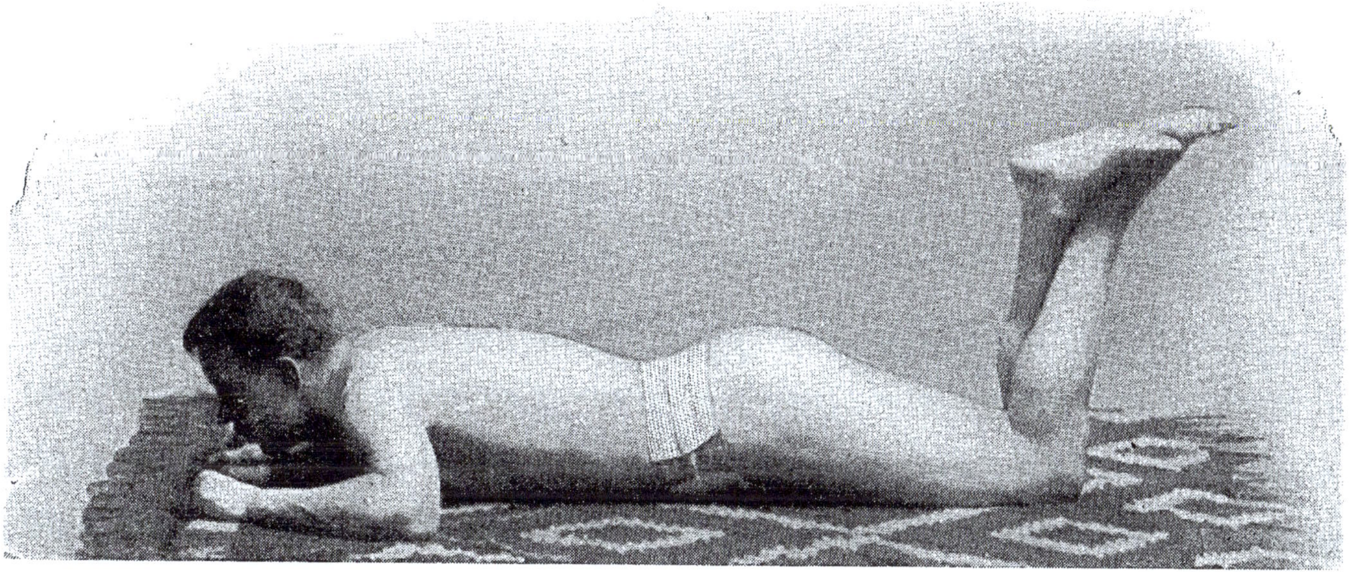

Exercise No. 12.

# CHAPTER XXXIII

## SPECIAL EXERCISES FOR VIGOR BUILDING

By no Means Difficult — Actively Use Nearly Every Muscle of the Body.

The exercises here illustrated are to be added to those preceding after becoming inured to the work. These exercises can be taken at night before retiring.

Continue each movement until slightly tired.

If you have an exerciser, or are already following some good system of exercise with the assistance of devices made for that purpose, the course with the apparatus can be used in their stead.

*Exercise No.* 13.—Assume position as per Fig. 13. Hold elbows at sides, and raise forearm up and down quickly forty to sixty times. Inhale deeply and full all during the exercise. Repeat three times. Next flex the muscles of arms, imagine you are lifting a very heavy weight, and bring hands up and down very slowly. This is for developing the arms.

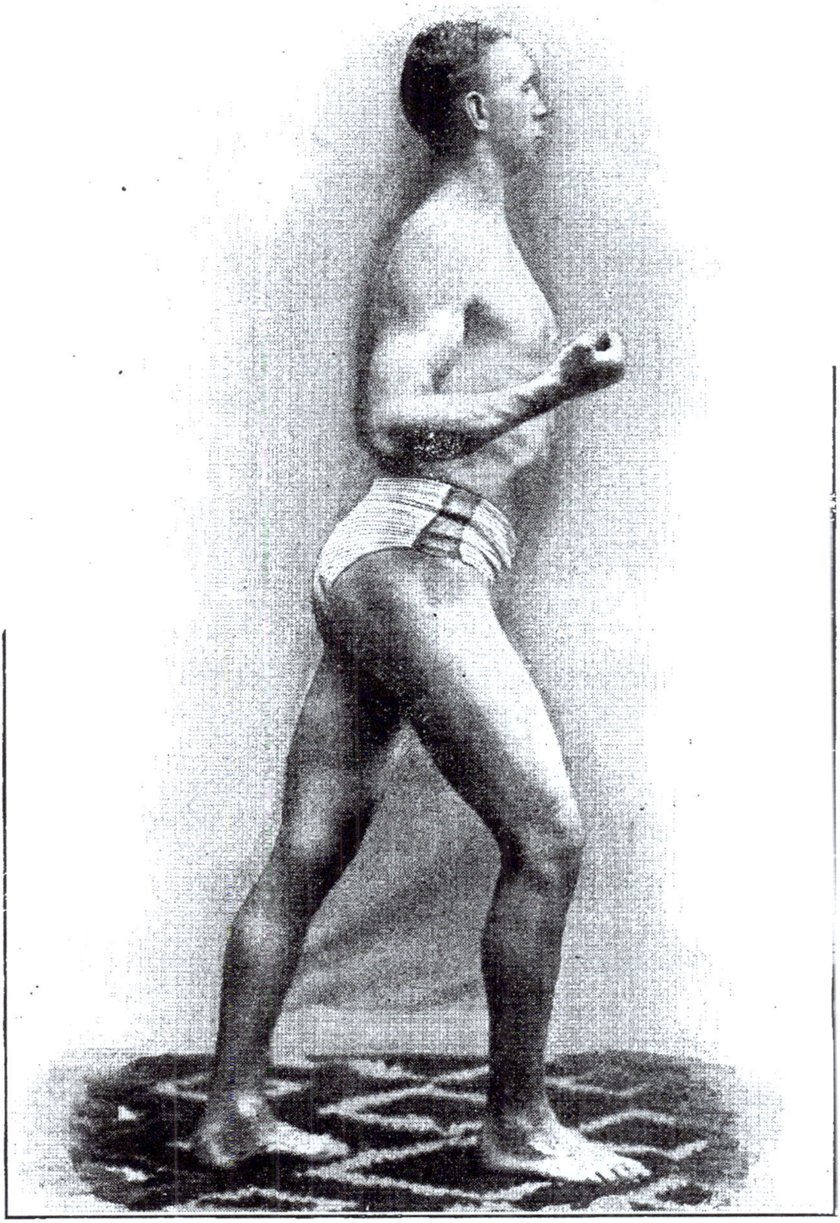

Exercise No. 13.

*Exercise No.* 14.—Assume position as in illustration No. 14. Draw deep inspiration, all you can, frequently during the exercise. Now keeping elbows rigid swing arms quick and strong, far backward and forward on a level with shoulders as long as you can conveniently retain the breath. Repeat until tired. For expanding the chest and increasing lung power.

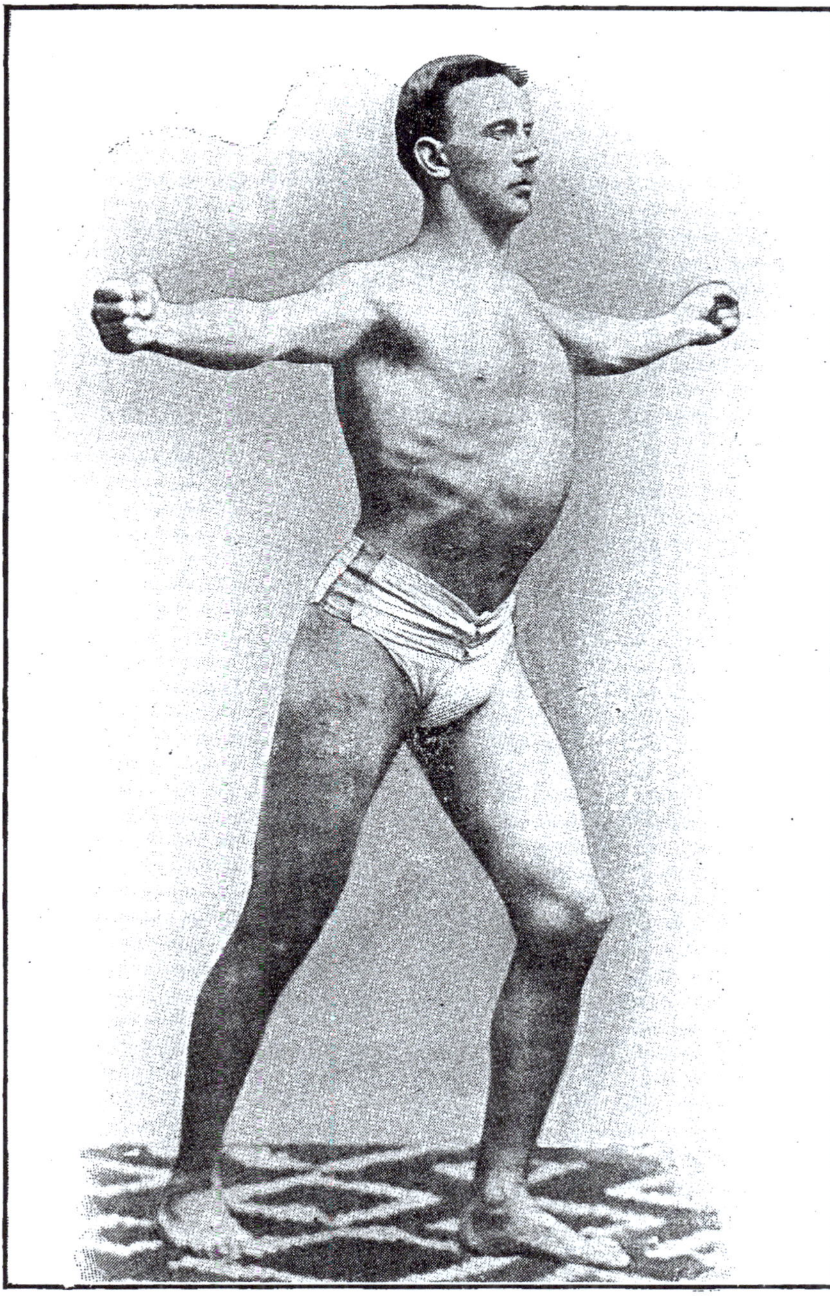

Exercise No. 14,

*Exercise No.* 15.—Stand erect, with feet far apart. Now touch the floor far to the right, as per illustration; then far to the left. Repeat exercise from ten to twenty times.

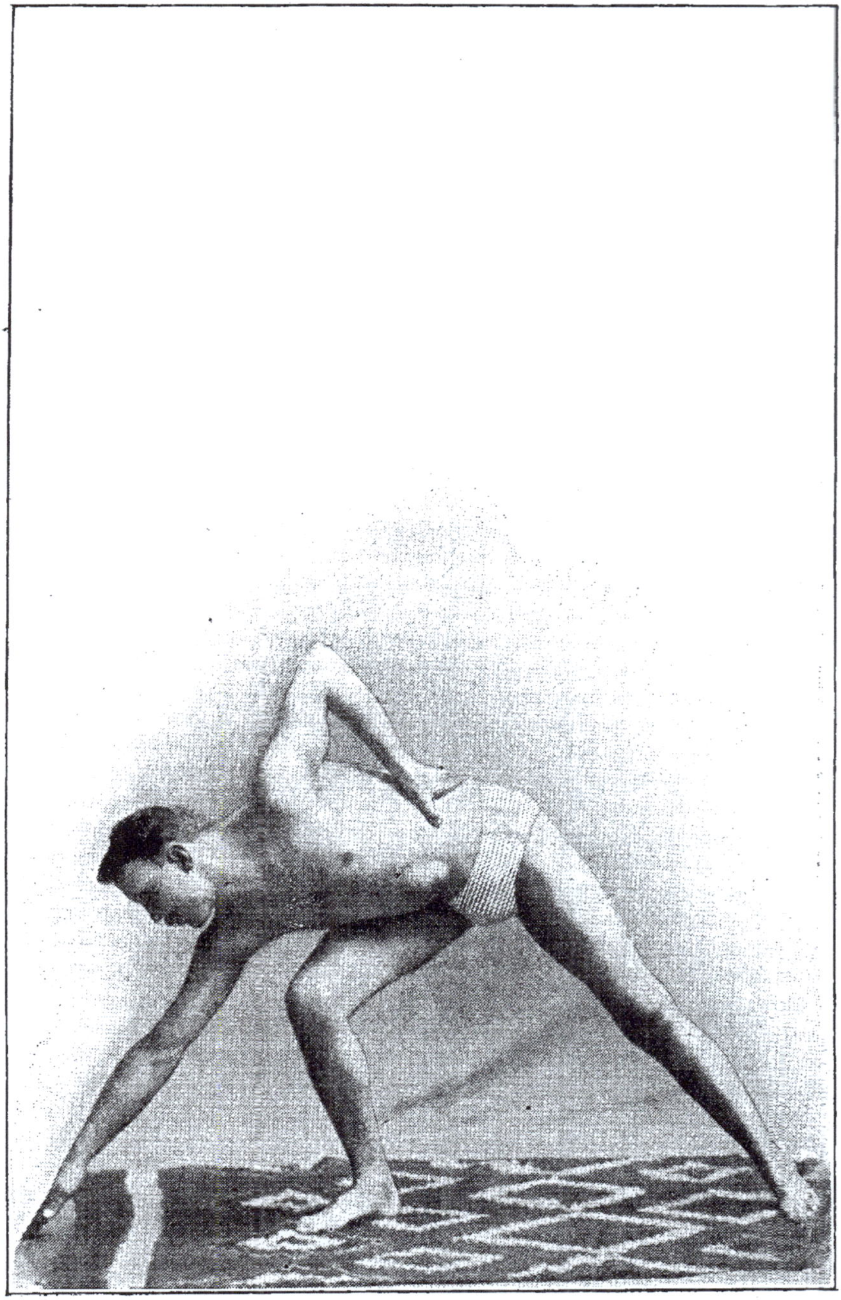

Exercise No. 15.

*Exercise No.* 16.—Assume position as in illustration No. 16. Keep knees very rigid, raise hands high as you can over head with elbows rigid, repeat from fifteen to twenty-five times. For strengthening the back.

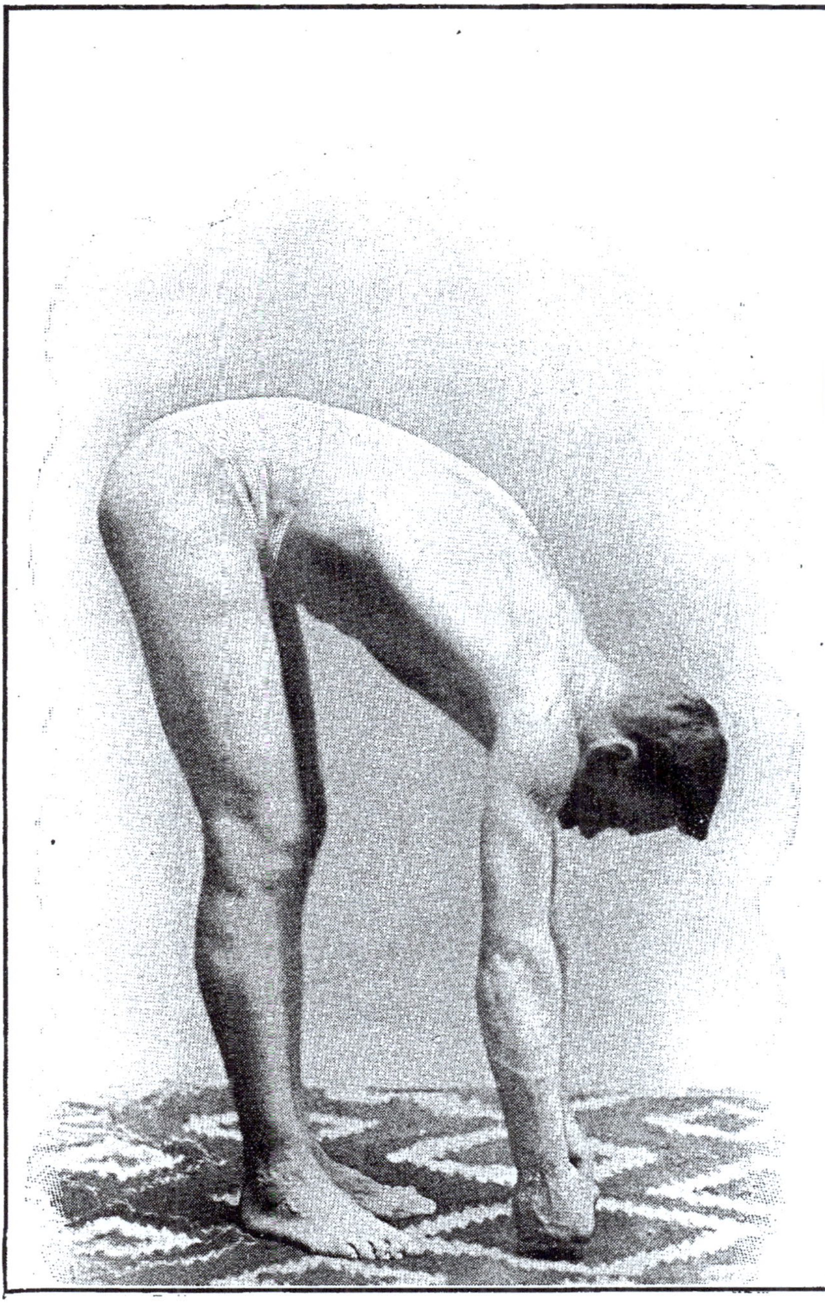

Exercise No. 16.

*Exercise No. 17.*—Brace yourself strongly as per illustration No. 17. Strike out hard and quick with right and left hands alternately, reaching as far as you can at each blow. Continue until tired. Count the number of blows each time you take this exercise to note how you are improving in endurance.

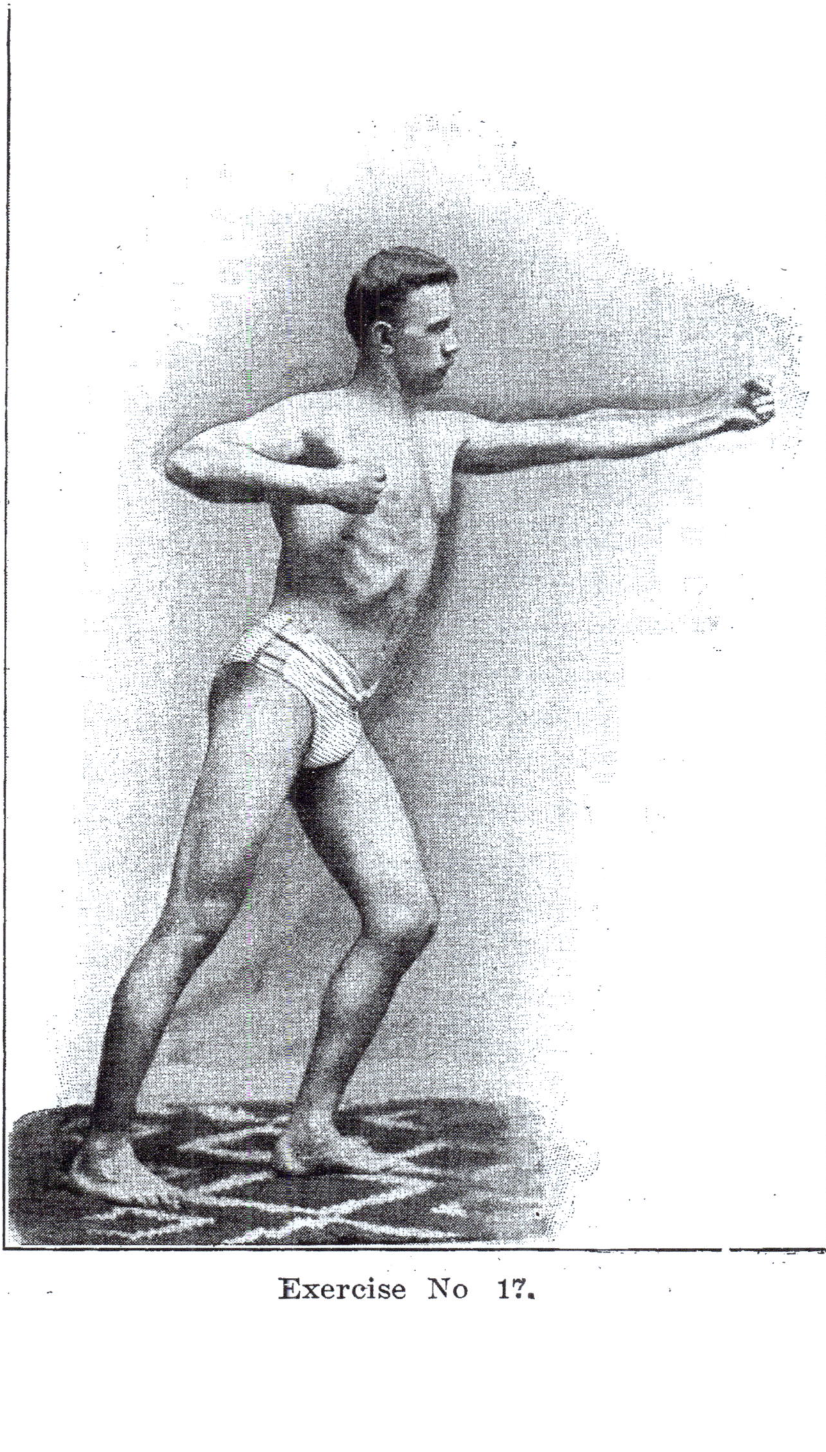

Exercise No 17.

# CHAPTER XXXIV

## WALKING AS A NERVE TONIC

It is One of the Most Effective Means of Restoring Poise to a Shattered Constitution.

Walking calls into action pretty nearly every muscle of the body and, under proper conditions, acts as a wholesome stimulant of the mental and nervous economies. For these reasons it is an ideal exercise and what is more, can be indulged in at all times and without cost except that of shoe leather.

The person to whom the benefits that can be derived from walking are unknown will be astounded if he will give it a thorough trial. Not walking as ordinarily understood, but walking for pleasure, for health.

No matter what sort of a contest an athlete may be training for, walking always constitutes an important part of the work. Trainers claim it hardens and develops the muscles and gives great powers of endurance to the one in training.

The walk for health must be taken in a different spirit from that which usually exists when it is taken for necessity. Put energy, life, action in every movement, every impulse of the muscles. Walk as though it was a privilege to do so and the result will be thorough enjoyment of the exercise. As to the distance to be covered to produce the best results, the writer advises that the walk be continued until there is a feeling of fatigue and that a comfortable seat would be much appreciated. Do not, under any circumstances, be too ambitious at first. It is far better to err on the side of moderation than of excess.

Gradually increase the distance as you become familiar with your strength and requirements.

Now come the instructions in reference

to walking from which, if observed, the greatest benefits in virility and health are to be derived.

At the beginning of your walk and for a short distance you must move rather slowly. Gradually increase your speed until you are traveling at a gait considered fast for you. As speed is increased begin to inhale deeply, always through the nose, expanding the chest to its greatest capacity from the abdominal region upward. While breathing thus deeply and fully make tense and hard the muscles of the arms and chest, bring the shoulders far back, while the abdominal region is fully expanded. Hold the shoulders in this position for a short time, and make endeavors to bring them still farther back. This exercise will tend to give proper carriage, and in connection with the special breathing, will cause you to realize that it is really and truly a "walk tonic." It is also a good idea to have some objective point for your walk and also to have a congenial companion with you. By these means a mental stimulus is established. If somebody accompanies you, however, beware of the temptation to race that will probably result. Remember that you are out for health and not for sprinting. This last will assuredly do you more harm than good if you indulge in it.

## CHAPTER XXXV

# DIET IN VIRILITY BUILDING

### Appropriate Food is Absolutely Essential to the Restoration of Vigor.

One of the most important principles of physical culture in acquiring strength and vitality is diet. Indeed, it may be called the fundamental principle, for no matter what steps may be taken for the purpose of attaining an ideal degree of physical health, unless you are subsisting on wholesome nourishing food, but little or no improvement in your condition can follow. Nothing indicates the importance of a properly arranged diet so clearly as the fact that it is possible for some to keep in approximately good health by careful attention to the quantity and character of the foods used, although but little care or time is given to exercise.

There has been a great deal learned recently about uncooked foods. The raw diet is becoming quite popular with a great number of people. The writer has lived on uncooked foods for months at a time with benefit. But after considerable experimenting of this character, he has about come to the conclusion that a combination of uncooked and cooked foods are best for the ordinary individual. Of course if you have studied the subject from a scientific standpoint, and understand yourself and your needs thoroughly, you might adopt an entirely uncooked diet. The list of appetizing foods that can be secured for a diet of this nature is almost unlimited.

If you are a meat eater, and do not feel that you can live without it, continue to use it, but I would strongly advise that you gradually lessen the quantity. In fact if you will experiment with your meals by gradually adding more uncooked and vegetarian dishes, you will be amazed to find how fast your craving for carnivorous food will decrease. Meats of every description will gradually be eliminated, if you allow yourself sufficient variety of edibles of the character mentioned. The writer's own experiences have been of this nature. For a long time he was in the habit of eating meat occasionally, and whenever he desired it, but gradually this appetite disappeared, and now it is only on rare occasions, when he cannot secure other kinds of foods that he tastes meat.

Therefore, my advice to a student who desires the greatest physical improvement would be to select cooked and uncooked foods from the long list of cereals, fruits, vegetables, eggs, milk, and nuts.

This chapter has been written not with the object of giving detailed information in reference to diet, but merely to emphasize its importance, for diet is an essential study in itself, and if the reader wishes a thorough familiarity with the subject, the writer would advise that he read some of the standard valuable books that treat of it. Do not read one only, and take its conclusions as absolute. Read several, and draw your own inferences therefrom. In this way your knowledge of diet becomes a part of you, and there is no necessity for time-wasting and tiresome reference to authorities when you are desirous of securing some particular point of information.

The statement is often quoted that "What is one man's food, is another man's poison." This it not true, though, as in the case of many false statements, one may find a grain of truth in it. Everyone knows the great power of imagination over the body. It has an equal power over the stomach and digestive forces. If one eats a food that he believes is harmful, he is continually on the lookout for signs to indicate that the expected trouble has begun, and in this way so centers his imagination and attention on the organs concerned that the expected symptoms are really induced by a sort of self-hypnotism.

Disguise any wholesome, nourishing food which the appetite normally craves, in such a manner that it resembles a viand that is supposed to result in injury to the person eating it, and in a great many cases unpleasant results will follow. On the other hand, the allegedly harmful food if in turn disguised will breed no ill effects.

Any change in diet should be slowly adopted. Do not suddenly stop eating foods that have agreed with you and start on an entirely different regimen. Feel your way, step by step, on any new diet you may choose to adopt.

Of course, we must admit that the digestive powers of individuals differ very materially. While one may be able to extract ample nourishment from a certain article of food, another may have some defect in his digestive organs, or possess gastric juices which will make it difficult to use this food to advantage. The importance therefore of developing and depending on a normal appetite in the selection of a satisfactory diet cannot be too strongly emphasized. An appetite of the description in question craves that special food element which is most needed at any or all times to nourish the body. Nearly all appetites are natural until made morbid by overeating, eating when not hungry, and other weakening practices. The longing for unwholesome foods in nearly every case indicates that the stomach is filled with a mass of fermented stuff which it is struggling to get rid of, and to do so it demands and obtains an excessive supply of gastric juice which in turn creates an unnatural appetite. The desire for alcoholic stimulants for instance, is always greatly increased if the stomach is suffering from repletion or from a series of meals eaten without appetite.

Nearly every authority on diet will advise one to eat slowly, but that does not mean to chew slowly. You can move your jaws as fast as desired. In fact, the faster one chews the more copiously the saliva flows, and consequently the more quickly the food becomes in a condition to be swallowed.

Masticate your food to a liquid before swallowing. Get all the enjoyment out of the process of eating that you possibly can. It is a sin against your body to eat without hunger. One of the most important digestive processes is brought into action by the keen enjoyment of food. It is not only the saliva but the gastric juice of the stomach that flows more freely when food is thoroughly enjoyed. But if no hunger is experienced when eating — if the food is bolted or washed down without appetite or relish — the digestive process is carried on with great difficulty and vigorous health is impossible in the presence of poor digestion and consequent poor nourishment.

Food eaten under such conditions is of absolutely no benefit. It had far better not be eaten at all. It simply gives the digestive organs that much more of a load to eliminate. No strength is gained from it. It lessens the muscular strength, for it takes the blood away from the muscles, that it may assist in the process of ridding the assimilative organs of the additional load that has been imposed upon them.

But you may say, " I must keep up my strength. I seem to be growing weaker all the time as it is and must eat, or I won't be able to walk." There you have it. The very means you have adopted to keep up your strength may be the cause of your weakness. Wait for an appetite if not hungry. Let this be an unfailing rule of your daily life. You cannot possibly enjoy vigorous health if this rule is not recognized and followed.

Yet others will say, " But I never grow hungry.

You need not worry one moment about that. Live on fruit juices from one to three days, and your appetite will be resurrected in all its youthful intensity, and with it will come renewed enjoyment, not only at the table but of everything in life. Food will then benefit you. It will be properly digested, and new life, new energy will thrill your nerves when purified rich blood begins to circulate through your veins.

If the diet is confined to foods that possess the needed elements of nourishment, it is not so much a question of what one eats, as it is of how much is eaten.

Eat what you can digest — what your appetite calls for; so much and no more.

When the food palls, when it ceases to be eaten with a keen relish, stop right there! Do not take another bite.

Avoid white flour and all articles of food made from it. No food for muscles, brain, or bones remains in this debased so-called superfine flour. All the important food elements have been removed with the bran. Not only is white flour greatly defective in nourishing qualities, but in many cases it is the cause of constipation. Eat whole wheat bread instead of white bread at your meals. The former is just what its name implies being made from the whole grain of wheat. No bran or any other nutritive part has been extracted from it. It is really a perfect food, for it contains in almost exact proportions the several elements necessary to properly nourish the body. See that this whole wheat flour is used instead of the white in every dish or edible requiring flour. You will find that this will make a great difference in your general condition almost from the first. You will feel better nourished, more energetic, healthier and happier in every way.

Cultivate an appetite for acid fruits. They can be recommended for use at all times.

Eat wholesome foods in general and avoid all fancy, highly-seasoned dishes.

If you care to experiment with your diet you will find that two meals per day will agree with you better than three. You may not be aware that when the stomach is overworked the digestive juices suffer in consequence, becoming weak and inefficient and unable to do their assimilative work properly. The result is that the food fails to create strength and energy. The remedy is to eat less and thus give the stomach a rest and allow it to store up gastric juice for the next meal.

Do not fail to bear in mind the necessity for doing that which will lead to your thorough enjoyment of food. Eat that which you feel you want, and leave all articles of food strictly alone if not relished.

Fasting for a few meals, or even for several days, will be found of great value in bringing about a normal condition of the digestive powers. But before attempting a long fast it would be well to make sure of your physical condition and the necessity for the proposed period of abstinence. In other words, " Be sure you are right, then go ahead."

## CHAPTER XXXVI

# PROPER BATHING INCREASES NERVE FORCE

Intelligently Used the Bath is One of the Most Effective of Tonics — Great Value of Dry Friction Baths.

Bathing nations are invariably strong nations. The Japanese for example are a people of scrupulous cleanliness, the daily bath being with them a matter of custom and indeed religion. The love of the Anglo-Saxon for his " tub " is proverbial. The " sweat-house " of our Indians before they were demoralized by contact with the pale-face was a tribal institution, and no savages were better endowed, physically or mentally, than they.

What is true of the nation is equally true of the individual. A clean skin is positively necessary to the development of the highest degree of physical and mental vigor. Not because dirt is in itself particularly injurious to the body, but because it clogs up the pores and lessens their activity, thus retaining in the system impurities and putting an undue strain on the other organs of elimination that should be assisted rather than hindered by the pores. A writer of some reputation on hygienic matters on one occasion maintained that the benefits of daily bathing were exaggerated. He stated truly that the skin was made up of millions of tiny scales that overlap each other like shingles on a roof top, and that as one scale was worn out, it was discarded and a new one underneath it took its place. But he claimed that an undue amount of bathing loosened these scales prematurely and so exposed the new scales before they were sufficiently hardened. He also asserted that the too frequent use of soap and hot water removed the natural oil of the skin, necessary as a lubricant, and that it had a tendency, therefore, to make it dry and harsh.

There is some amount of truth in his remarks in as far as his statement in reference to the too frequent use of hot water and soap is concerned. A hot bath should not be taken over two or three times per week in spite of the fact that alleged authorities on the subject claim that a daily hot bath is necessary to ideal cleanliness.

The assertion that the body cleans itself by casting off scales as they become dried is true to an extent and if the body were exposed to the air in the same way as is that of any animal, on would not suffer very much if he never took a bath. Yet it is well to note that animals and birds find keen enjoyment in baths when there occurs an opportunity for them to take them. But as long as we wear clothing which shuts out the air and which absorbs the impurities cast off by the body, so long will the necessity for frequent bathing remain. The activity of the pores of the skin in the way indicated, renders the bath — tepid or cold — an imperative element in the acquirement of perfect health. The importance of this principle cannot be over-estimated.

Unquestionably one can bathe too much. One can eat too much bread. Exercise can be taken too much. In fact, no matter how beneficial anything may be, it can be the means of producing injury if used to excess.

Yet while it may be possible to bathe too much, the writer believes there is but little danger to be feared from that source.

The accumulation on the skin of stale perspiration and other impure matter eliminated through the pores makes a hot bath with plenty of soap desirable two or perhaps three times per week.

When treating yourself for sexual weaknesses of any kind the morning exercise should always be followed by a friction bath. This consists of brushing the skin all over with two soft bristle brushes, or rubbing it thoroughly with a dry rough towel. When the brushes are used they should be drawn back and forth over every part of the skin until it is pink from the circulation induced by the friction.

The skin will naturally be very tender in the beginning, though it will soon become inured to the treatment and the brushes can then be used for a considerable time without inconvenience or discomfort.

The effect of this friction bath on the appearance of the skin is wonderful. In a short time it will become as smooth and soft as velvet, and absolutely free from all pimples and blotches, especially if a rational system of diet is being simultaneously followed.

Usually it is of advantage to follow this dry friction with a cold sitz bath, of about one minute's duration. Such a bath consists of the immersion in water of the hips only, and it can be taken most conveniently in a tub made for the purpose. A small ordinary tub, or washtub will serve, or a large bathtub will do if one is muscular enough to place the heels on end and then lower the body in the water, the soles of the feet remaining unimmersed. After sitting in the water about one minute, wet the body all over and dry quickly with a rough towel.

If there are no conveniences for taking this bath, wet the body with cold water, and stoop over a basin until you can bathe the private parts also.

While the friction bath may be discontinued after a recovery of vigor, yet it will be found a powerful tonic in aiding the system to retain normal vigor, and for that reason should by no means be neglected.

Many shrink from the use of cold water, and believe that they cannot become accustomed to its use. This can easily be done without any shock worth mentioning if the proper process is adopted. Accustom

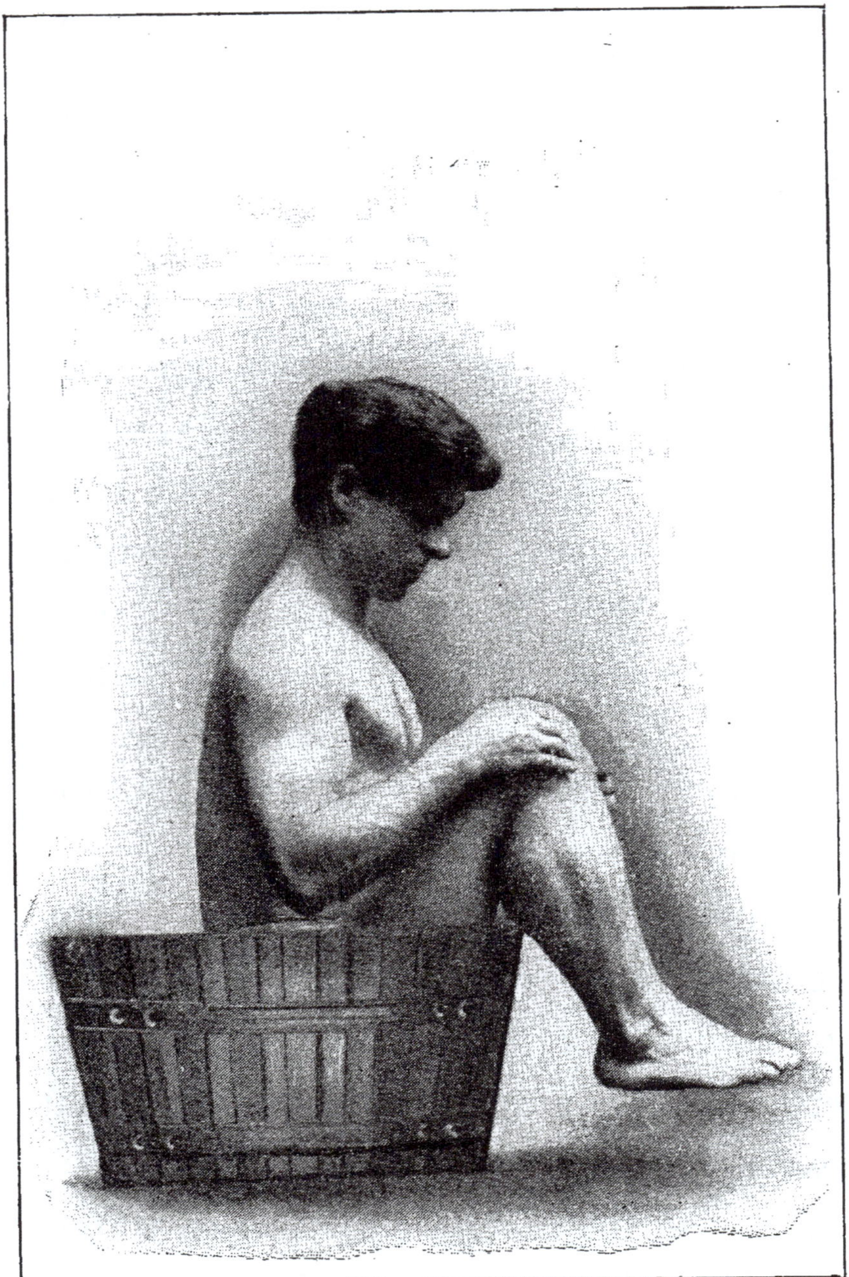

Showing how a sitz bath can be taken in an ordinary tub.

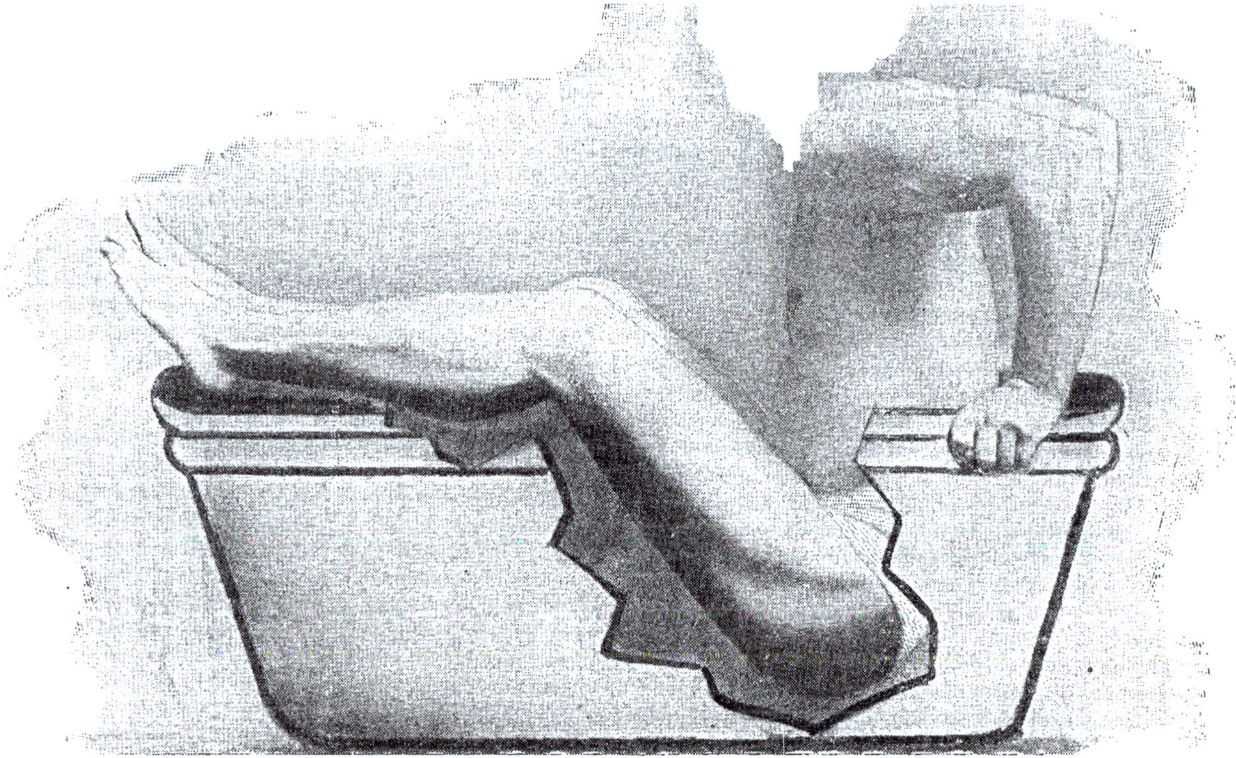

Another method of taking a cold sitz bath. The bath tub is not as convenient as a tub made expressly for the purpose, but will do if one is sufficiently strong enough to lower body by the arms.

yourself to use it gradually. Begin with tepid water and make it a little colder each day. Many, however, find not the slightest difficulty in taking cold baths right from the first provided the baths immediately follow the exercises and friction bath by which the circulation is so awakened that the body is well able to resist the shock of the water and the subsequent effects are exceedingly pleasant.

If chilly after a cold bath, exercise until warm. This will insure you against any ill-effects whatever.

Do not forget that if the entire surface of the body was varnished over, death would ensue in a few hours, because of the accumulation of impurities that usually find their outlet through the pores and also because we inhale or absorb oxygen through the pores as well as through the lungs. Nothing could prove the necessity for regular bathing more emphatically than that one fact. Of course, there are many who bathe only on rare occasions, and a few who never bathe at all, but unless they live an extraordinary clean life dietetically, which means the avoidance of meats and many cooked foods and wear but little clothing they are the kind who are satisfied with merely existing and are not good to meet physically or in other ways. They do not live in the true sense of the word. They eke out a nauseous existence. Their presence outrages our senses of smell and sight and they imbue us with a sense of repulsion and disgust.

To really live, to feel the energy and power of superb health pulsating in every nerve, and vein, and muscle, to be thrilled with a sense of the power of opulent life, every physical function must be in perfect working order, and this cannot be brought about unless the pores of the skin are kept open and active by regular and appropriate bathing.

# CHAPTER XXXVII

## PURE AIR AND MANLY VIGOR

You Cannot Hope for Perfect Health Unless Insured Plenty of Unpolluted Oxygen.

A famous authority on hygienic matters has written that men live more on air than they do on food. This is an emphatic and at first glance, startling statement. Yet it is scientifically correct nevertheless.

Air is an essential to the life of all created beings and pure air is one of the chief factors in the acquisition and maintenance of health. One can exist on bad air, it is true, but to exist does not necessarily mean living. The average individual seems to imagine that this is of little importance, whereas it has a tremendous influence on his general health. There was never a more serious blunder made by a humanity that is prone to blunders. There is food in air. Oxygen is a food. It is just as necessary, in fact far more necessary to life than any other element which enters into the constituents of the body. A man can live for sixty days without solid food, he can live for several days without water, but he can not live five minutes without oxygen. Did you ever think of that? Consider the importance and enormous value of pure air, rich in oxygen and determine that you will take pains to have your lungs liberally supplied with it. Remember that you cannot acquire or retain sexual or any kind of power for any length of time if this necessity for pure air is not recognized and acted upon.

Are you afraid of draughts? Well hurry up and rid yourself of this ridiculous fear. It has dug premature graves for thousands. Did you ever notice that the more a man feared draughts the more colds he seemed to acquire, and the weaker he seemed to become, while the careless man who gave but little attention to them was healthful, and rarely, if ever, had a cold? This was because his lungs were fed with a plentiful supply of oxygen at all times, and the thousands of little pores all over his body also had a chance to exhale their foulness and inhale pure air.

Do not waste your time by taking the treatment advised here unless you can forthwith make up your mind to supply your body with unpolluted air in plenty. To do this decide that you will not sleep in a badly ventilated room. Open the windows wide — the wider the better. Cultivate a love for a current of the outside atmosphere. Breathe it deeply at all times; bathe your body in it. It means life, health and strength. It is the greatest tonic in the world. It attacks and kills the impurities of the body, it assists in the digestive process and it greatly accelerates the process of elimination constantly going on through the pores as well as the lungs.

Of course, if you are accustomed to smothering yourself with clothing and sleeping with hermetically sealed windows do not adopt the other extreme all of a sudden. Your body is like a plant made delicate by being kept from the bracing influences of sun and air. If such a plant is exposed to breezes and the direct rays of the sun without preparation, it is liable to suffer from the change. But expose it a short time the first day, a little more the next day, and so on, and finally it will become vigorous and hardy, capable of bearing any amount of exposure. By coddling and too extreme care, breathing the atmosphere of inclosed rooms over and over again, until it is actually foetid with the poisons emanating from the lungs, and by shutting out draughts and sunlight, one can easily deteriorate into a fragile human plant, and one will remain such, delicate and weak as long as that which created the condition is allowed to exist unchanged.

Turn over a new leaf at once. Pure air — not rotten air — was the intention of Nature. Inclosed air becomes debilitating and disease-breeding. Remember too that a sickly plant has no claim to vitality and neither will you as long as you deny your body the fuel of vitality — oxygen.

The writer takes an air bath daily. Such a bath is necesary to the acquirement and retainment of the highest degree of health. Take your exercise in your own room, nude, with the windows moderately open at first, and open them wider each day. Build the internal fire! Make the blood glow throughout your body while in this nude state by vigorous movements and deep breathing.

The writer follows this practice in the coldest of weather. Often when the thermometer registered below zero he has exercised nude in his room with the windows wide open and with the wind blowing full upon him. Strange as it may seem to the average reader, such exercise in a nippingly cold atmosphere is most enjoyable after a few movements have been made. Of course, the transposition from a warm bed to the chilly room gives one a momentary shock, but this passes away in a very short time and there follows a feeling of exhilaration, or physical exaltation, which is hard to describe, so delightful is it.

The more that colds are feared and the more attempts that are made to protect oneself against them by coddling, the more colds one will acquire. This is an unfailing rule, and no one who has given the matter any attention can question its truth or have difficulty in explaining the cause. The direct contact of the skin with air stimulates the action of the pores on account of the circulation of the blood in the capillaries being accelerated by their friction with the air in motion, together with the direct absorption of oxygen by the pores themselves.

This is the explanation of the wonderfully beneficial results that follow on the use of air baths as described. Again let it be said that the importance of allowing the surface of the body to come into direct contact with the air as much as possible cannot be too strongly emphasized. Air "massage" as described, is a most important factor in the building of a vigorous, healthy, nervous and muscular organism. Especially is it beneficial to the nervous system, having a quieting and strengthening effect thereon.

Begin at once to cultivate a love for fresh pure air. It will almost immediately increase the virile powers of your manhood, and you will reap rewards from a habit of this kind that could not be purchased in any other way by all the wealth in Christendom.

Oxygen is life, and full, opulent life is

the basis of magnificent manhood. Per-contra, lack of oxygen, or impure air lowers the vitalities and saps manhood.

"Whenever foul air is breathed, the blood is not properly purified, and the body cannot be properly nourished. Enough poisonous and waste matter to spoil half a barrel of water is thrown out by the lungs at every breath."—*E. Bouton.*

# CHAPTER XXXVIII

## INFLUENCE OF MENTAL ATTITUDE

### Train Your Mind to Dominate Your Body and Good Will Surely Follow.

The body is or should be the subject and instrument of the mind. A departure from this principle is pretty apt to result in trouble or unhappiness of some sort or other. It will, for instance, be found that that which we call sin consists of the ignoring of the promptings of the higher nature or mind, in order to pander to the desires or demands of the lower or the body. And sin and misery are identical terms. "Gratify my lusts," whispers the body. "Pollute not me or yourself by the flesh," commands the mind. If the body's wishes are gratified it is emboldened by its mutiny, grows stronger at each successive act of rebellion until the man is under its dominion altogether.

On the other hand and under the majority of conditions, the power of the mind over its shell of flesh and bone is never absolutely lost and it can moreover produce apparent miracles if proper means are used to invoke its latent possibilities. It is certain that the sickness or health of the body do, to an extent, reflect the condition of the mind. It is also certain that if the mind can be persuaded that neither it or the body are ill, both assume an attitude of health and vice versa. Suggestive therapeutics are based upon this phenomenon and in Christian science, we find it given first place as a remedial agency, upon which the founders of the sect have built an elaborate system of treatment which depends entirely on the faith of the patient in accepting the dictum that " There is no Evil only Good " and that consequently there does not really exist either ill health or misery of any sort. This is magnifying the power of mind over body to a tremendous extent, but the importance of the underlying principle must not be overlooked or denied on that account.

Thousands of healthy human beings go through life with an unshakable belief in their minds that they are suffering from some insidious disease, when their ailment really exists only in their imagination. Such a mental condition, if continued is fairly sure to produce actual disease of the type dreaded. The morbid conditions that produce the belief must be discouraged as much as possible, and exercise, cheerful companionship, lots of cold water and common sense are excellent things to use in this connection. Remember that disease or weakness is unnatural, and that the body, if given an opportunity, will actually cure itself. No matter how serious may be your alleged or otherwise trouble, vow that you will make the necessary efforts to secure health, and that you do not merely hope to secure it, but that you intend to see that you do so in one way or another. Use your will power. Put out of mind any doubt or suggestion that any other results than those desired can possibly follow, and you will be amazed at the influence that this clearing of your mental atmosphere will have toward bringing about rapid recovery.

"Every young man who desires to remain strong, or to regain his physical, intellectual and moral powers, should have an absorbing purpose in life. Live with an aim, and let that aim be high. The man who aims at the sun will shoot higher than the man who aims at the earth. If you do not build a few castles in the air, you never will own any that are built on the earth. Devote yourself with untiring diligence to some department of work. Determine what is to be your life-purpose, and devote yourself absorbingly to its attainment.

Do not be contented with mediocrity. Rise above the masses. Attain to eminence. Be thorough from the very beginning. Be diligent. And if you will thus devote yourself to the untiring attainment of some worthy purpose, there can be no question in regard to your future acquisition, your life will be worth something."—*Sylvanus Stall, D.D.*

This influence of mind over body is of especial importance in all sexual troubles. Ailments of that nature seem to cast a gloom over the victim that is difficult to dissipate. But do not allow it to eucompass you! Fight it as you would a human enemy, for it is an enemy of the worst and should be treated as such. Keep it as far from you as possible. Be pleasant with yourself. Make yourself good company for yourself and for others. Cultivate a smiling countenance. If your features are acquiring a wan, chronic, worried expression, command them to smile occasionally and after a time they will smile often. Think of something funny as often as possible. Look at the humorous side of life. The best time to joke is when misfortune or death stares you in the face. Anyway, why fear death? You only have to die once. It usually takes more courage to live than it does to die. Anybody can die! That is simple; but there are occasions when it takes real bravery and determination to live.

Let your first efforts toward building for yourself the virile powers of superb manhood be spent in the coincident cultivation of a cheerful countenance, and a sanguine mind. Stop worrying at once. It is a waste of vital strength — it is a strain on nerves and muscles — it keeps you in a tense, rigid condition as though you were constantly on the alert for fear of some terrible calamity. In this state it is impossible for you to grow strong and hearty while you are certainly growing weak and puny. Do the best you can, and then say to yourself: " I don't care what happens. I've done my duty. I'm not at fault," and then you will find that the best will happen.

The most severe form of criticism is self criticism. One can stand the criticism of others, but the flaying of oneself by oneself is the most terrible of all criticisms to a conscientious person. Therefore, see that you have no cause for self-blame, and then stop your self-inflicted torture which makes you a nuisance to yourself and to others.

Do not forget that you can invoke mental influences to your moral and physical undoing and mental influences to your salvation. Some psychologists assert that all our actions are the outcome of self-suggestion or self-hypnosis. The " objective " consciousness tells the " subjective " consciousness what is to be done or left undone and its commands are obeyed to the letter. " I intend going to Boston to-morrow," says one part of yourself to another part of yourself and acting on the suggestion you as a whole, pack up and go. "I want to wake to-morrow at six o'clock" impresses one part of yourself on another part of yourself and sure enough no matter how soundly you are sleeping or what you are dreaming about, you open your eyes on the stroke of the hour.

"I will think good thoughts and do nothing but honest, healthy acts," says the man of clean life and high purpose. And the suggestion rules his career.

"Now I'm going to imagine last night's good time all over again," chuckles the rouè and his passion-steeped being gladly accepts the suggestion, and so he revels in soul-soiling thoughts and dreams.

"From hence on I intend — no, I AM — going to live decently and uprightly, giving my body its meed of wholesome food and proper exercise, and my mentality the food upon which it too can thrive and the care that it too deserves," declares the young man whose eyes have been opened to the sin and folly of a fast life.

And the dominated part of his nature hears and obeys the order of the dominant, and the erstwhile weak, wretched, sin-stained youth becomes by force of his self-suggestion the MAN that he declares he will be.

Reader, try the experiment. Say to yourself, " I will " or " I will not," and note the results.

# CHAPTER XXXIX

## ABBREVIATED GENERAL INSTRUCTIONS.

### A Daily Régime for General Development of All Bodily Powers.

Determine that you are going to profit by these instructions.

Make a compact with yourself to observe them faithfully.

Rise when you awake if you have had from seven to nine hours' sleep.

Take the exercises prescribed while nude.

Follow these exercises with a dry friction bath.

Then take a cold sitz bath to be followed by wetting all of the body.

Eat only two meals daily.

If you eat three daily meals make your breakfast of fruits.

Don't eat too heartily at night.

Eat your last meal from three to five hours before retiring.

Sometime during the day take a long walk, with many deep breathing exercises.

Don't waste nervous force in useless hurry.

Don't worry!

After becoming inured to the exercises, take the special course of exercises in chapter XXXIII just before retiring if not too fatigued.

Don't cover yourself too heavily when in bed.

Open your windows widely.

Whether married or single occupy a bed by yourself.

Retire early enough to allow yourself having from seven to nine hours of sleep.

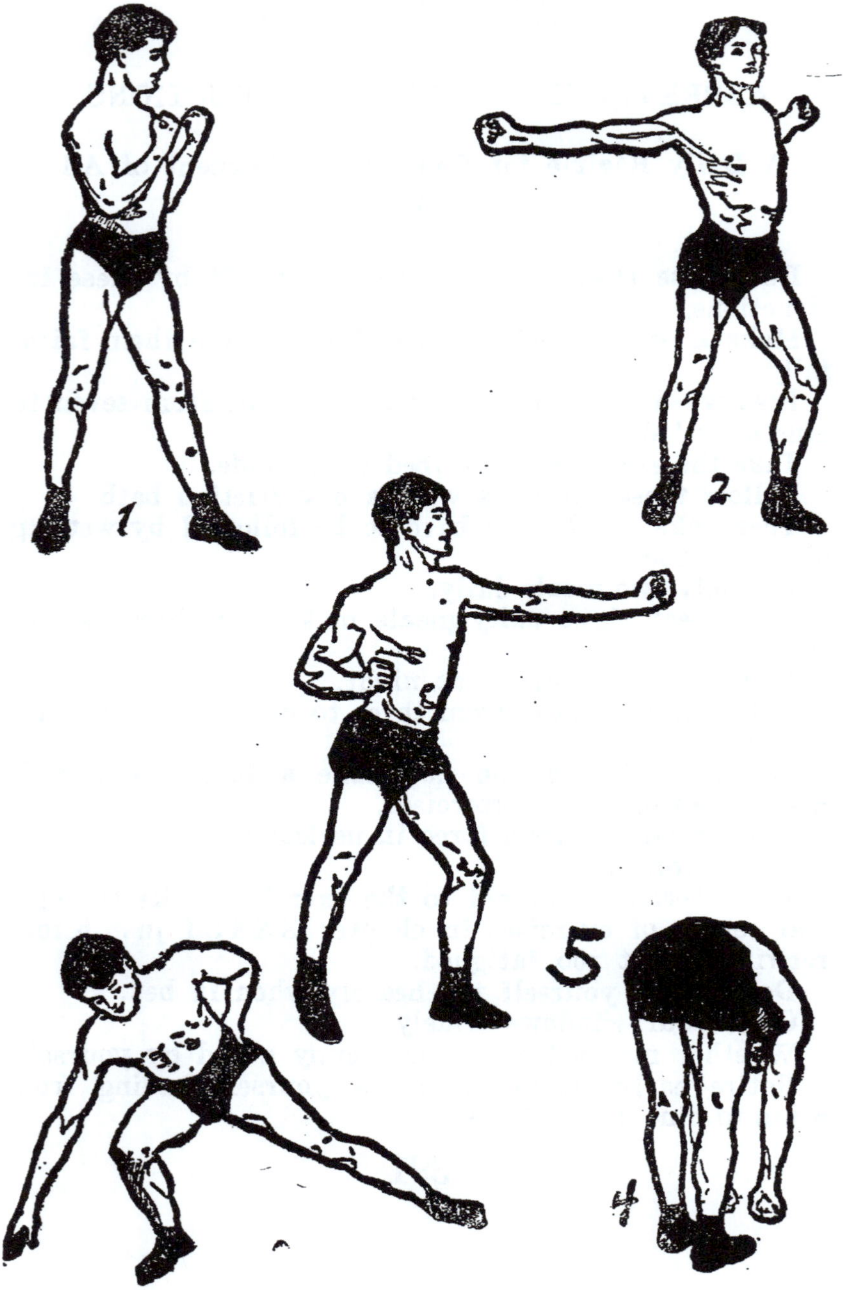


Résumé of Special Exercises for Vigor Building. Especially Good for Developing the Chest, Shoulders. Back and Arms.

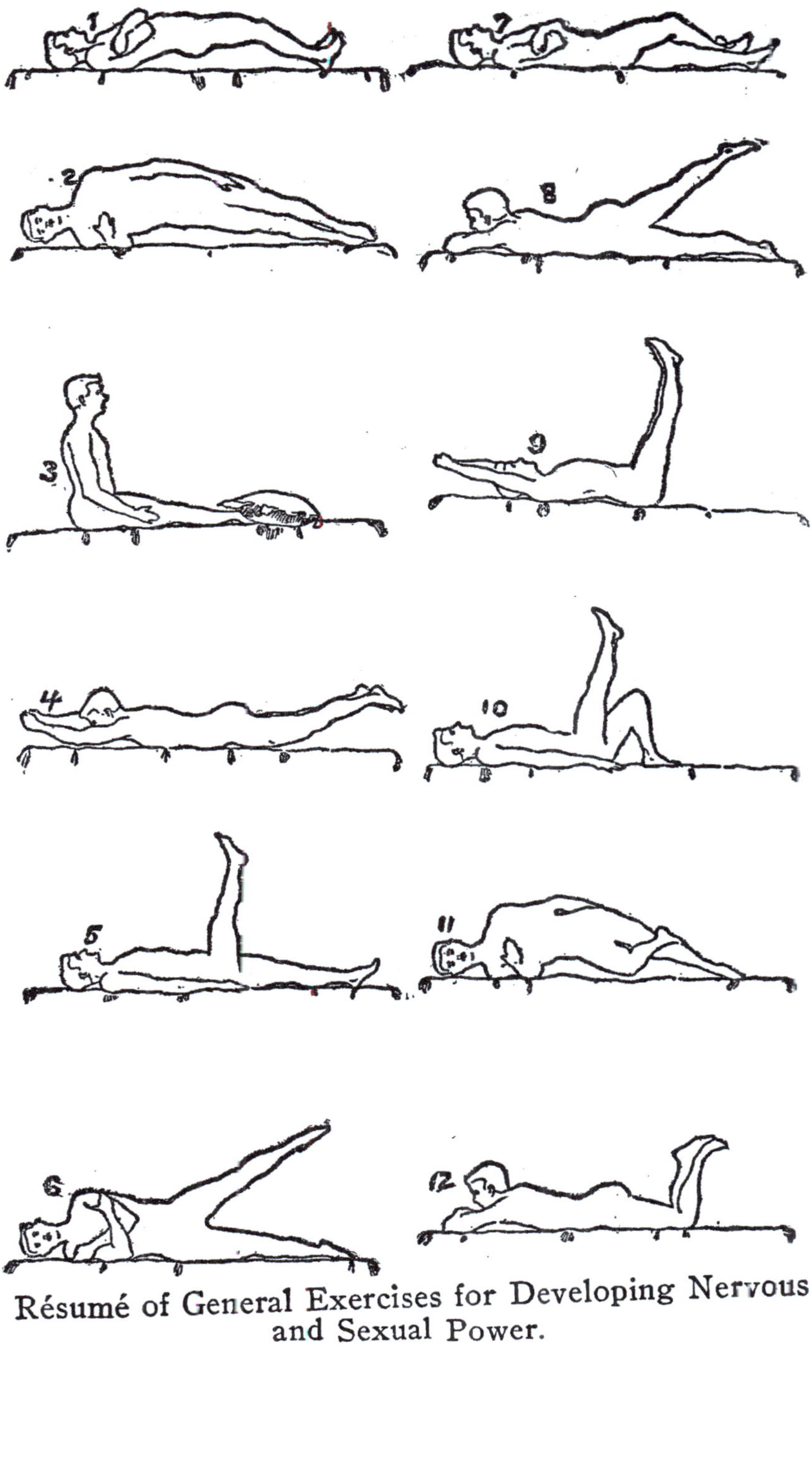

Résumé of General Exercises for Developing Nervous and Sexual Power.

# Building of Vital Power

## Deep Breathing and a Complete System for Strengthening the Heart, Lungs, Stomach, and all the Great Vital Organs. Profusely Illustrated.

Every man, woman and child needs great vitality, for that means strong internal organs. It means the possession of that strength which is absolutely essential to the acquirement and retainment of superb health. This book tells you how to increase the vital powers of all the important organs. It is plain and concise. If you care not specially for muscles, but want to feel at all times exhilarated with superbundant health, secure this book and follow the plain directions contained therein.

CHAPTER I.—What is Vital Power?
CHAPTER II.—Vital Power Depends on Functional Vigor.
CHAPTER III.—Pure Blood and Vitality.
CHAPTER IV.—Organs of Digestion, Circulation and Respiration.
CHAPTER V.—Building Vital Power with Long Walks.
CHAPTER VI.—Vast Importance of Water.
CHAPTER VII.—Increasing Digestive and Assimilative Power.
CHAPTER VIII.—How a Powerful Stomach May Be Acquired.
CHAPTER IX.—The Heart Made Powerful.
CHAPTER X.—Developing Great Lung Power.
CHAPTER XI.—Pure Air of Utmost Importance.
CHAPTER XII Illustrated suggestions for perfect ventilation.
CHAPTER XIII.—Erroneous Methods of Breathing.
CHAPTER XIV.—Deep Breathing Exercises.
CHAPTER XV.—How an inexpensive lung tester can be made at home (illustrated).
CHAPTER XVI.—Breathing and Muscular Exercises Combined (illustrated).
CHAPTER XVII.—Sun and Air Baths Vitalize Body.
CHAPTER XVIII.—Importance of the skin, kidneys, lower bowels and lungs.
CHAPTER XIX.—Perverted ideas in regard to clothing.
CHAPTER XX.—Restful Sleep Powerful Means of Building Vital Force.
CHAPTER XXI.—Mental Attitude Important Factor.
CHAPTER XXII.—Dry Friction Bath Exhilarating Skin Tonic. Profusely illustrated.
CHAPTER XXIII.—Importance of Constant Bathing.
CHAPTER XXIV.—Diseases of Kidneys. How caused. General treatment.
CHAPTER XXV.—Constipation Destroys Vitality.
CHAPTER XXVI —How to Remedy Constipation.
CHAPTER XXVII.—Exercises for Remedying Constipation.
CHAPTER XXVIII.—Summing up Results.
CHAPTER XXIX.—General Regime for Daily Practice.

Bound in cloth, post-paid. $1.00

**PHYSICAL CULTURE PUB. CO.,**

# STRONG EYES

**A Valuable and Interesting Book**

**By BERNARR MACFADDEN**

---

A SYSTEM OF TREATMENT WHEREBY WEAK EYES MAY BE MADE STRONG AND SPECTACLES DISCARDED

---

## CONTENTS

CHAPTER I.—Eyes Most Important of Human Organs of Sense. The Mechanism and Mystery of Sight.

CHAPTER II.—The Physical Causes of Beautiful Eyes. Elusiveness of Definition.

CHAPTER III.—Strong Eyes Main Factor in Personal Magnetism. The Limitations of the Blind and the Weak-sighted.

CHAPTER IV.—Dull Eyes; The Cause and Remedy. Absurdity of Looking for a Local cause or of Seeking for Local Remedies.

CHAPTER V.—How Weak Eyes May Be Strengthened. Evils of Present Education of School-children.

CHAPTER VI.—Crippled Eyes; How Caused. The Eyes that are Made so.

CHAPTER VII.—Diseased Eyes; How to Treat Them. Inflammation and its Treatment.

CHAPTER VIII.—Constitutional Treatment for Weak Eyes. Out-of-Door Exercise. Diet.

CHAPTER IX.—How Eyes are Improved by Massaging Them. How the Eye may be Massaged with the Fingers.

CHAPTER X.—Illustrated System For Exercising Eyes.

CHAPTER XI.—How the Valuable Eye Bath is Taken. Shown by Illustration.

CHAPTER XII.—Special Exercises for Improving Eyesight.

CHAPTER XIII.—Exercises for Constitutional Treatment.

Bound in cloth, postpaid, $1.00.

# Physical Culture for Baby

By MARGUERITE MACFADDEN
and BERNARR MACFADDEN

***Profusely and Handsomely Illustrated***

This book tells all about Babies. It tells you why Babies are cross, why they are good. It tells you how to make your Baby fine, strong and healthy. In fact, there is nothing about Babies that a mother should know which will not be found in this invaluable work. It answers all the important questions of mothers relating to Babyhood from the moment of birth until Childhood.

## CONTENTS

# STRENGTH FROM EATING.

BY BERNARR MACFADDEN.

## How and what to eat and drink to develop Suppleness, Strength and Beauty of Body.

Muscular exercise develops strength, *providing nourishing foods are furnished.* Knowledge of the elements of which all foods are composed is absolutely essential in order to develop strong and beautiful muscles.

This book teaches you not only what to eat and drink, but how to eat. It gives you information which the author has collected from fifteen years of study and experimentation.

You spend part of every day in eating. Do you know how and what to eat to build increased strength? If not, this book will tell you. Read it! Think as you read, and if the plain truths it contains do not cause you to make radical changes in your diet, return the book and get your money back.

TITLES OF CHAPTERS.

Appetite. Mastication. Process of Digestion. Air a Food. Three-Meal Plan. Two-Meal Plan. One-Meal Plan. Necessity of Pure Water. Meat, or Mixed Diet. Vegetarian Diet. Raw Diet. Cooking of Foods. Food and Occupation. Over-eating. Alcoholic Liquors. Alcohol is not a Food. Drinking at Meals. Coffee and Tea. White Bread Curse. Elements of Foods. Muscle Making Elements Fattening Elements. Analysis of the various foods made from wheat. Oats and Other Grains Vegetables. Dairy-Products. Fruits. Meats. Nuts. Fish.

*Bound in Cloth, prepaid, for $1.00.*

# Power and Beauty of Superb Womanhood

BY BERNARR MACFADDEN.
Assisted by Medical and Other Authorities.

**How Developed to the Highest Degree of Attainable Perfection.—How These Grand Powers are Lost and How They May be Fully Regained.**

You cannot afford to be without this new book. It is worth its weight in gold to any woman with brains enough to read, think and act. It will enable her to make something of herself. It will enable her to develop her highest attainable degree of beauty and power of body. It will save many thousands of dollars in doctor's bills. Every book is sold with a guarantee to return the money to every dissatisfied purchaser.

CONTENTS.

**Superb Womanhood.** Its great value. **Present Physical Condition of Woman.** Physical wrecks everywhere. Physical condition of women of the stage and of those in society. **Causes of Wrecked Womanhood.** Abnormal and weakening influences begin in babyhood. Overfeeding, excessive clothing, bad air, fear of sunlight. Fearful results of prudishness. **The Curse of Prudishness.** Ignorance not innocence. Plain duty of mothers and fathers. Must daughters secure their knowledge from vulgar associates, or from pure sources? Marriage a physical union, founded on physical attraction. Instinct the only right guide in 'falling in love." Influences before marriage prevent the development of this instinct. Depraved idea of modern marriage. **Corsets.** Origin of the use of this devise. Courtesans at the time of the degeneracy of Greece introduced it. False standard of beauty perpetuates it. Delicacy no longer a sign of beauty. **Corsets Weaken Digestion! Destroy Beauty. Increase Natural Size of Waist! Age Women Prematurely and Destroy Womanhood.** Downward pressure of corsets misplaces, weakens and destroys the organs of sex. **Operations that are Crimes.** The knife recommended for every abnormal manifestation produced by impure blood. A cure possible in every case without a dangerous and unsexing operation. **Can Wrecked Womanhood be Reclaimed?** Exercise, breathing, proper diet, etc., the great remedies. The great importance of proper foods. Four important rules. **How to fast to produce results. How Exercise Beautifies the Body. Photographs of Defective Figures. Exercises for Developing Suppleness and Symmetry.** A special system of exercises illustrated by photographs. **Exercises for Bust Development. Exercises for Remedying Physical Defects. Exercises for Remedying Female Weaknesses. Natural Treatment of Female Weaknesses.** Symptoms, cause and natural home remedy for Congested or Inflamed Ovaries— Ovarian and Womb Tumor— Suppressed Menstruation— Painful Menstruation—Sterility—Displacement of Womb, etc. **Childbirth made Painless by Exercise.** Great benefit that can be derived from air baths. **Bathing and Water Treatment. Infallible Remedy for Constipation.** Special exercises for remedying the trouble, illustrated. **Massage as a Beautifier. Friction Baths. How to Obtain A Perfect Complexion.**

*Bound in Cloth, prepaid, for $1.00.*

SD - #0012 - 130824 - C0 - 229/152/23 - PB - 9780282488086 - Gloss Lamination